Ultrasound in Rheumatology

Qasim Akram · Subhasis Basu
Editors

Ultrasound in Rheumatology

A Practical Guide for Diagnosis

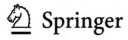 Springer

Editors
Qasim Akram
Stockport NHS Foundation Trust
Stockport, Greater Manchester, UK

Subhasis Basu
Radiology Department
Wrightington Hospital
Wigan, UK

ISBN 978-3-030-68661-1   ISBN 978-3-030-68659-8   (eBook)
https://doi.org/10.1007/978-3-030-68659-8

This Springer imprint is published by the registered company Springer Nature Switzerland AG
The registered company address is: Gewerbestrasse 11, 6330 Cham, Switzerland

May this book be an inspiration to my new-born son Haaris Mikaeel Akram
To my Wife, Parents and Akram family for their continuous love, motivation and support

Akram

Dedicated to my wife Sudipta and family for their endless support, sacrifice and continuous inspiration

Subhasis

Foreword

Since the beginning of the twenty-first century, point-of-care musculoskeletal ultrasound has been progressively and firmly incorporated into rheumatological practice as an extension of clinical assessment and as an essential aid to optimise the diagnostic process and the therapeutic decisions in the wide spectrum of rheumatic diseases, from inflammatory arthritis, microcrystalline arthropathies, osteoarthritis, connective tissue diseases or vasculitis to soft tissue syndromes. Moreover, ultrasound is a bedside tool for improving the accuracy and safety of musculoskeletal injections and biopsies.

Nowadays, ultrasound allows us not only to accurately and finely image musculoskeletal structures and tissues involved in adult and paediatric rheumatic diseases but also to evaluate other tissues involved in immune-mediated diseases that are readily accessible to ultrasound like the lung, vessels or salivary glands.

In addition to technological advances, many advantages of ultrasound have made its growing implementation possible in the clinical setting, such as accessibility, relatively low cost, absence of invasiveness, real time and dynamic nature, and great acceptance by patients, children or adults. In addition to this and of utmost importance, ultrasound allows the scanning of all peripheral joints as many times as required at the time of consultation as well as providing an immediate correlation between imaging and clinical findings, which undoubtedly enhances both for the benefit of the patients.

In our time, in which rheumatology should aspire to excellence, ultrasound has become an essential part of our portfolio of services to society and health system stakeholders, and therefore, a mandatory part of our educational programme for young and future rheumatologists. As ultrasound is the most operator-dependent imaging modality, mainly because of the intrinsic real-time nature of image acquisition, high-quality training is extremely important to ensure skilled and safe point-of-care use of this imaging modality by rheumatologists. A solid knowledge of sectional anatomy, physics and technology, scanning method, pattern of normal and pathological tissues, artefacts and definitions and diagnostic criteria for abnormalities are all necessary to properly perform ultrasound. Thus, it is the obligation of senior rheumatologists to provide new generations with instruments and methods to learn ultrasound in a feasible and efficient way, compatible and consistent with the many other training requirements of the specialty.

This book offers a comprehensive but at the same time simple and friendly bedside educational tool in the fundamentals, ultrasound scanning technique and diagnostic skills of the musculoskeletal system and other anatomical structures involved in rheumatic diseases for all those colleagues, especially the youngest, who decide to start in the exciting world of rheumatological ultrasound.

So, I think this book should be used as a friendly companion to increase enjoyment, learning and good practice.

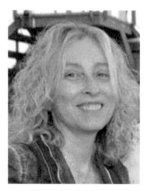

Esperanza Naredo, M.D., Ph.D.
Department of Rheumatology and
Joint and Bone Research Unit
Hospital Fundación Jiménez Díaz
Madrid, Spain

Acknowledgements

We would like to thank all the contributors who have made this book possible.

Their time, hard work and passion for this project have been greatly appreciated especially during the unprecedented COVID-19 situation. We would like to thank the contributors for adhering to the deadlines given to them.

Special mentions must go to Dr. Najmul Huq, Consultant Musculoskeletal Radiologist and Dr. Eilidh McGowan at Stockport NHS Foundation Trust for their helping in putting together hand and wrist and foot and ankle chapters. Dr. Jay Panchal at Wrightington Hospital has helped with both the shoulder and hip chapters as well as Mr. Dean Eckersley and Mr. Niall Rowlands. Dr. Riccardo Terrenzi and Dr. Iustina Janta have been extremely helpful in providing material for the pathology figures at the end of each chapter. Dr. M. Takhreem has worked tirelessly with Unzag Designs, based in India, to ensure the accuracy of the anatomical figures.

Dr. Akram would like to thank Dr. Chandini Rao and Dr. Marwan Bukhari, Consultant Rheumatologists, for supporting and encouraging him to pursue ultrasound fellowship training overseas whilst a specialist trainee.

Professor Naredo has been a constant mentor and support throughout my training to not only become a competent ultrasound practitioner but also have a vision for and challenge boundaries of ultrasound use in rheumatology. Dr. Akram is very grateful for this.

Introduction

In recent times, the usefulness of Ultrasound (US) has become more important in rheumatological diseases. US is safe, relatively cheap and most importantly allows a high standard of imaging, without the need for contrast, and can be performed at the bedside. Rheumatologists have started to believe its capability as a significant adjunct to the standard consultation process comprising of the clinical history and physical examination.

US offers an interesting and tangible evaluation of anatomical structures that are affected by rheumatological diseases and has enhanced our understanding of the pathophysiology of certain diseases and their processes. It is a powerful tool for patients to understand their disease especially in the modern world of fast-moving technology and instant gratification.

As an adjunct to the usual history taking and physical examination, it has a high sensitivity for picking up synovitis in early rheumatological disease (as high as MRI) and enables early treatment to be initiated which improves both patient satisfaction and disease outcomes.

US has a high pick-up rate for erosions, which can be a predictor for aggressive disease and can accurately detect entheseal abnormalities which is a feature of Spondyloarthropathy. US also detects and can be helpful in differentiating degenerative disease from inflammatory arthritis as well as crystal arthritides. Colour doppler can detect the characteristic 'halo sign', which reflects vessel wall oedema in large vessel vasculitis and may prevent the need for a more invasive temporal artery biopsy. US is useful for showing abnormalities of the intima-media complex, which is another feature of large vessel vasculitis.

US is also accurate at demonstrating the morphology of the salivary glands in Sjogren's and can detect changes of interstitial fibrosis in lung disease. Ultrasound detects needles as being hyperechoic and can accurately depict the path of the needle into the target region, i.e. real time as well as providing important information of the target area beforehand and highlighting the most suitable angle, depth and direction of the needle. This ensures accurate and safe use of injections minimising any adverse effects including lipoatrophy and inadvertent damage to any nearby structures.

We believe that every modern Rheumatologist should be well equipped at being able to perform an ultrasound examination at the point of care and in fact, should be considered as being the Rheumatologists stethoscope or extended finger. Some have described this as a stethoscope. In fact, it is more accurate, and we prefer to avoid that analogy.

Barriers to training, especially in the UK and US, have meant a lack of uptake in most rheumatological practices in comparison to Europe, for example, as well as some traditional approaches suggesting that point-of-care ultrasound may not have a place in the rheumatologist's office.

To be able to perform ultrasound safely and effectively, considerable time and experience are necessary, and some form of assessment/accreditation should be undertaken to reflect this. This is important for commissioning and safe training of others.

From a practical level, a good anatomical knowledge is mandatory in addition to a knowledge of sono-anatomy which is usually seen in cross section and a knowledge of rheumatological disease processes.

This book has been created to assist in the practical development of ultrasound skills for the rheumatologist. Although it is not an anatomy book, useful anatomical diagrams have been provided to help better visualise the structure being examined. These are anatomical diagrams which we have used to teach and lecture on ultrasound. Ideal probe position and ideal image acquisition are detailed, and the authors envisage that this should be used as such and at the bedside. Typical pathological images have been documented at the end of each chapter demonstrating synovitis, tenosynovitis, erosions, osteophytes and crystal arthritides in the upper and lower limb sections. Large vessel vasculitis, Sjogren's syndrome and interstitial lung disease on ultrasound are shown in the relevant chapters.

We hope you enjoy this book as much as we enjoyed producing it. Good luck on your ultrasound journey.

Yours sincerely
Dr. Qasim Akram

Contents

Editors and Contributors

About the Editors

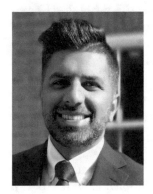

Dr. Qasim Akram Consultant Rheumatologist, Stockport NHS Foundation Trust, Stockport, Greater Manchester, UK. Dr. Akram is a hugely enthusiastic practitioner and teacher of musculoskeletal ultrasound in rheumatology. He is a Consultant Rheumatologist and General Physician based in Manchester, UK. Dr. Akram is very much a pioneer of ultrasound training in the UK and has completed a highly specialised musculoskeletal ultrasound fellowship at a Centre of Excellence at Gregorio Hospital Maranon, Madrid under the guidance of Prof. Naredo. Dr. Akram was the first rheumatologist to carry out a dedicated ultrasound fellowship in Europe during his specialty training, paving the way for other rheumatologists to follow. His vision is for every modern-day rheumatologist to be able to use ultrasound. He currently leads the Stockport Early Inflammatory Arthritis Ultrasound Clinic, which is one of the first of its kind in Greater Manchester. He is a EULAR Ultrasound instructor and teaches ultrasound on a local, regional and national level to other Consultant Rheumatologists, Specialty Trainees and Allied Health Professionals. He is the lead instructor for the North West Rheumatology Ultrasound Network. His main clinical research interests are focussed on the use of ultrasound in rheumatoid arthritis, psoriatic arthritis/spondyloarthropathies, crystal arthritis and large vessel vasculitis.

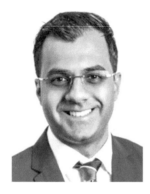

Dr. Subhasis Basu Consultant Musculoskeletal Radiologist, Wrightington Hospital, Wigan, Greater Manchester, UK. Dr. Basu is a Consultant Musculoskeletal Radiologist based at Wrightington Hospital, Wigan, an Orthopaedic Centre of Excellence. Dr. Basu has completed a highly prestigious Advanced Musculoskeletal and Sports Imaging Fellowship at Chelsea & Westminster Hospital, London. Dr. Basu has a particular interest in musculoskeletal ultrasound in rheumatology and works closely with rheumatologists to provide rapid diagnostic and therapeutic services including inflammatory arthritis and degenerative diseases. Dr. Basu is one of the leading 'up and coming' MSK radiologists in the UK and is a hugely popular teacher. He teaches regularly at national courses including the Oxford Radiology Course and has a further interest in education and research through his established University roles as well as multiple journal and book chapter publications on various aspects of MSK Radiology.

Contributors

Andreas P. Diamantopoulos, M.D., Ph.D., MPH Martina Hansens Hospital, Bærum, Norway.

Andreas P. Diamantopoulos works as a Consultant in Rheumatology at the Department of Rheumatology at the Martina Hansens Hospital in Oslo, Norway. He holds a Ph.D. from the Norwegian University of Science and Technology (NTNU) in Trondheim, Norway, and a Master's in Public Health from the University of California at Berkeley, USA.

Dr. Diamantopoulos has a deep and long-standing interest in musculoskeletal and vascular ultrasound. He is the founder and director of the first International Ultrasound Workshop in Large Vessel Vasculitis in Kristiansand, Norway, where he established one of the first fast track vasculitis and musculoskeletal ultrasound clinics. He is a member of the EULAR/ACR working group on Polymyalgia Rheumatica, the European Vasculitis Study Group (EUVAS), the OMERACT group on ultrasound in LVV. For his research activity, he has been rewarded the award for the best clinical abstract in EULAR 2013 in Madrid and two times the travel award of the Japanese College of Rheumatology.

His current research is focusing on the use of ultrasound as a diagnostic and follow-up tool in large vessel vasculitides.

Dr. Anne Bull Haaversen, M.D., Martina Hansens Hospital, Bærum, Norway.

Anne Bull Haaversen is a Consultant in Rheumatology at the Department of Rheumatology at the Martina Hansens Hospital in Oslo, Norway. Dr. Haaversen is specialised in vascular ultrasound and her current research is focussing on the use of vascular ultrasound in the diagnostics of Giant cell arteritis. She teaches on a regular basis including International Ultrasound Workshops in Large Vessel Vasculitis.

Dr. Iustina Janta Consultant Rheumatologist, University Hospital Valladolid, Spain.

Dr. Iustina Janta is a Consultant Rheumatologist at University Hospital Valladolid, Spain performing musculoskeletal ultrasound in daily clinical practice as well as teaching peers and other trainee rheumatologists.

She has a special interest in musculoskeletal ultrasound in inflammatory and autoimmune diseases (rheumatoid arthritis, spondyloarthropathies, crystal induces arthritis) and salivary glands in Sjogren syndrome.

She has participated as a trainer in National and International (EULAR) musculoskeletal ultrasound courses (adults and paediatrics) since 2012. She had published several peer-reviewed articles on ultrasound in rheumatic diseases and participated in a recent EULAR task force for standardised procedures for Ultrasound Imaging in Rheumatology.

Dr. Juan Carlos Nieto Gonzales Consultant Rheumatologist, Hospital Gregorio Maranon, Madrid, Spain.

Dr. Nieto González is a Consultant Rheumatologist based in Hospital Gregorio Maranon, Madrid, Spain, and Associate Professor of the Universidad Complutense de Madrid.

He has completed both EFSUMB and EULAR accreditation (Level 2) in musculoskeletal (MSK) ultrasound and is an enthusiastic and popular Instructor. He is a Professor of Paediatric MSK Ultrasound for the Spanish Society of Rheumatology. He teaches fellows and is an organiser of the national Salivary Gland Ultrasound course at Hospital Gregorio Marañón.

Dr. Maria Takhreem Anaesthetist (Specialist Trainee), Wrightington Hospital, Wigan, Greater Manchester, UK.

Dr. Maria Takhreem is a final-year Specialist Trainee in Anaesthetics currently working in Wrightington Hospital, Wigan, an Orthopaedic Centre of Excellence. She is currently training in advanced regional block techniques (with ultrasound) for both upper and lower limb surgery.

She has a particular interest in ultrasound physics and including its application to day-to-day practise in her role as an anaesthetist. She is a very keen and enthusiastic teacher and is regularly involved in training both undergraduates and postgraduates.

Mr. Stuart Wildman Advanced Practice Physiotherapist, Consultant Musculoskeletal Sonographer and Honorary Lecturer at Brunel University London. Director of The Ultrasound Site Ltd.

Stuart is an Advanced Practice Physiotherapist and Consultant MSK Sonographer working in the NHS in London. He has an interesting working week, dividing his time between Radiology and Physiotherapy, where he performs both diagnostic ultrasound and ultrasound guided injections.

He is very passionate about the use of ultrasound amongst health professionals and is committed to teaching. He has founded The Brunel University Post Graduate Certificate in MSK Ultrasound Programme alongside other colleagues. He is the Director of The Ultrasound Site, an ultrasound-based educational platform offering a wide variety of courses and mentorship programmes for allied health professionals and doctors.

He is regularly invited to speak at conferences in the UK and abroad and is very active on social media through The Ultrasound Site.

Essentials of Ultrasound for Practical Scanning

M. Takhreem and Q. Akram

What is Ultrasound and How Does It Work?

Ultrasound refers to sound waves that are above the acoustic spectrum, which in the human ear is usually at a frequency of 20–20,000 Hz (or 20 kHz). Every 1,000 Hz equates to 1 kHz. Some animal can hear up to 100,000 Hz (or 100 kHz). Medical ultrasound equipment ranges from a frequency of 1 MHz (1,000,000) to 50 MHz (50,000,000) [1].

Frequency refers to the number of cycles per unit of time i.e. one cycle per second is 1 Hz. On the other hand, wavelength is the distance between each cycle of sound [1].

Frequency and Wavelength are inversely related. For example, as the frequency increases the wavelength is reduced and as the frequency is lowered the wavelength is increased (Fig. 1) [1, 2].

Ultrasonic waves with a higher frequency tend to penetrate less than a lower frequency waves. The resolution will, however, increase with increased frequency . Conversely, a lower frequency means a higher wavelength of sound waves and a better penetration . However, this will result in a lower resolution. Relating to this in practical scanning in rheumatology, most joints i.e. hands and feet are located superficially so will require a higher frequency meaning less penetration and shorter wavelengths but a higher resolution [1, 2].

Attenuation is a reduction in power and intensity of sound as it travels through tissue. Higher frequencies attenuate or absorbed faster than lower frequencies (i.e. less tissue penetration) (Fig. 2) [3].

M. Takhreem
Wrightington Hospital, Wigan, Greater Manchester, UK

Q. Akram (✉)
Stockport NHS Foundation Trust, Stockport, Greater Manchester, UK
e-mail: qasim.akram.qa@gmail.com

1

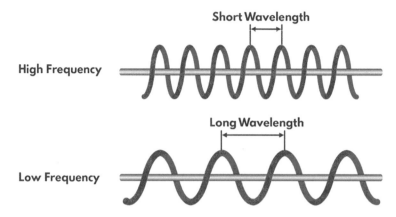

Fig. 1 Diagram showing relationship between frequency and wavelength

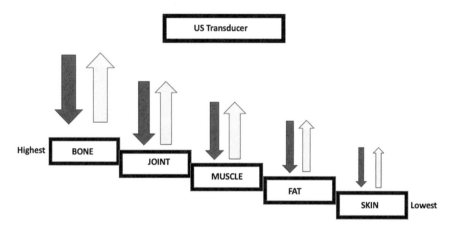

Fig. 2 Acoustic impedance of different tissues

Acoustic impedance, resistance encountered by US waves as pass through a tissue, is related to the density of the material and the speed of sound in the material. The greater the difference in impedance between tissues, the more sound will be reflected rather than transmitted. Acoustic impedance is slow in air, higher in muscle and even higher in bone so sound beams do not penetrate bone at all hence the high reflectivity. Liquids such as blood and synovial fluid do not reflect sound waves (Fig. 2) [2].

The acoustic interface refers to the boundary between two different tissues. Ultrasound waves that are emitted are reflected at the interface of two different tissues. The greater the difference in tissue density the more reflective the boundary will be while similar densities pass easily through the tissues. The amount of reflection and transmission is dependent on speed of the sound waves and the specific acoustic impedance [2].

Fig. 3 Gel standoff required on ultrasound probe for accurate image acquisition

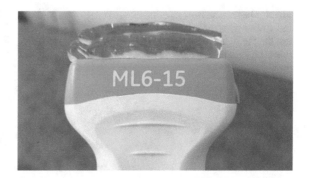

Fig. 4 Diagram showing gel standoff and good image acquistion

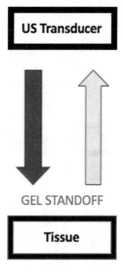

Due to there being an interface between skin and air, large amounts of gel have to be applied as a medium (Figs. 3 and 4). If the surface of an object is flat and no air is present between source and object, almost all the US waves transmitted from the transducer will be reflected at right angles from the object (Fig. 5). The returning ultrasound waves are detected by transducer which contains crystals of lead creating an electric current. The electronic potential is then converted into an ultrasound image by the computer and interpreted by the operator (Fig. 6) [2].

Modes Used in Ultrasound?

B mode or grey scale is the precursor of grey scale ultrasound and is limited by defining boundaries of structures and differentiating fluid from solid. It cannot differentiate between fibrous tissue and active synovitis.

Fig. 5 Diagram showing
inadequate gel stand off
resulting in sound wave being
reflected at a right angle from
the object

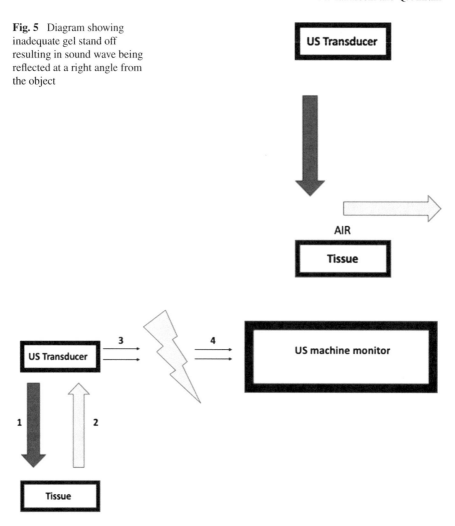

Fig. 6 Diagram showing image acquistion- US transducer sends sound waves towards the object [1] and they are reflected back to the tranducer from the tissue [2] and then converted into an electrical signal [3] which displays as an US image on the monitor [4]

Doppler is the detection of movement by measuring a frequency shift in the returned echo (Figs. 7 and 8).

Power doppler (PD) ultrasound displays the doppler power in colour. Power doppler uses the strength of a returned sound wave from anything that is moving to give the position and brightness. It increases the sensitivity of the machine to small vessels and slow blood flow which is present in hyperaemia in inflamed tissues. Hence, its usefulness to detect active inflammation in synovial joints [3, 4].

The doppler principle states that sound waves increase in frequency when they reflect from objects moving towards the transducer and then decrease when they

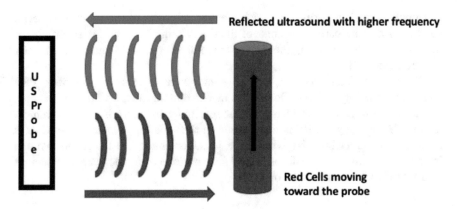

Fig. 7 Doppler principles- red cells moving towards the probe

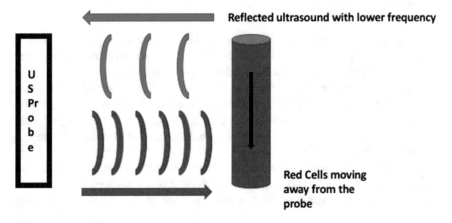

Fig. 8 Doppler principles with red cells moving away from the probe

reflect from objects moving away from the transducer (Figs. 7 and 8). As with grey scale, if the frequency is higher it gives a more detailed image of vessels but less penetration. A lower frequency gives a deeper penetration but a poor resolution. The gain determines the sensitivity to flow and increasing the gain will the increase the sensitivity of the signal returning from the machine. A lower gain reduces any noise and motion artefacts (see below) but also the sensitivity. Thus, to obtain the most accurate power doppler image, the gain should be increased till background noise is detectable and then reduce it gradually until it has gone [4, 5].

Colour doppler combines doppler principles with real time imaging and creates a colour signal. This signal indicates direction of blood flow. Red cells on the screen indicate movement towards the probe and blue is away. In addition, colour doppler uses the amount of frequency shift from anything that is moving to determine the speed of movement (Fig. 8) [4, 5].

Doppler signal is formed by a combination of power of the sound wave sent, number of moving particles, depth of the tissue being assessed i.e. superficial or deep joint, the PRF and amplification of the returned signal (PD gain) and the box size/frame rate [4].

Higher PRF filters remove low flow and there is less noise. Lower PRF increases sensitivity to lower flow, gives machine more time, also time for deeper signal to return. Lower PRF has a higher sensitivity but there is more movement artefact. Using a lower PRF is more useful in rheumatology where slower flow is detectable. A larger box size when assessing doppler reduces the frame rate and impact on sensitivity and reduces risk of false positive from artefact above such as mirror or reverberation (see below) [5].

What Are the Common Ultrasound Artefacts and How to Reduce Them?

Artefacts in US can be described as echoes which either by depth , direction or amplitude do not correspond to a real tissue or target. An awareness of common artefacts is helpful to interpret ultrasound scans accurately [6].

Anisotropy is the term used for the ultrasound artefact encountered in tendons, nerves and muscles. This is due to a scattering of the beam which is not perpendicular to the surface. These returning waves are not fully captured by the probe and so appear dark. The tendon may appear hypoechoic and this create a false impression of disease (Fig. 9) [6].

Acoustic shadow occurs when the ultrasound beam is reflected when it hits a highly reflective surface such as bone or calcifications. This creates a dark area beneath it such as when calcific tendonitis is seen in the rotator cuff tendons (Fig. 10) [2, 6].

Fig. 9 Anisotropy due to scattering of the beam because the transducer is not perpendicular to the tissue

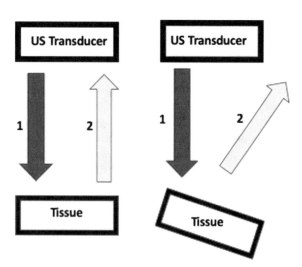

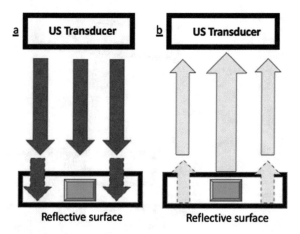

Fig. 10 Acoustic shadowing due to a highly reflective surface. In (a) the middle (red) arrow shows the beam not able to penetrate the reflective surface. This returns back to the transducer in (b) creating a highly reflective signal (middle large yellow arrow). There is no signal below the reflective surface creating a dark area below it. You can see that signal either side is trasmitted correctly creating a normal image (smaller red and yellow arrows)

Fig. 11 Reverberation artefact seen when waves hit an object such as a needle. It can actually help guide accurate placement of ultrasound guided injections

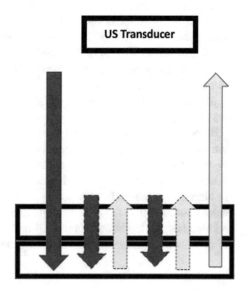

Reverberation is a key phenomenon of the beam bouncing back and forth between transducer and object giving small echoes. This is seen when a needle is introduced in tissue whilst performing ultrasound (Fig. 11) [5, 6].

Refraction occurs due to the transducer sending signals at an oblique angle rather than perpendicular as the ultrasound waves crosses the edge of tissues of different densities. This propagated signal is lost and image clarity is reduced. Remember that conventional setting assume the returning signal as though

Fig. 12 Refraction of sound beams

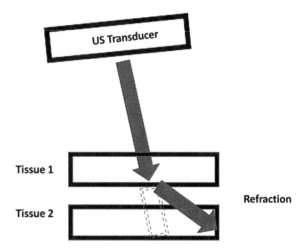

travelling in a straight line. To avoid this the probe must be kept as close as possible to 90° (Fig. 12) [5, 6].

Random noise is seen as a colour foci randomly in the image. Random noise can be avoided by lowering the gain just below setting that has little or no noise as described above. Motion artefact is detected by any movement of the patient, machine or probe. This is limited by keeping the patient in a comfortable position and avoiding any unnecessary movements and fixing the ultrasound machine and the examiner must avoid any movements of resting arm. Mirror artefact is caused by any highly reflective surfaces like bone and doppler image is prone to such. Doppler mirror show false flow below a bone surface [5, 6].

Blooming artefact is colour beyond vessel wall making vessels looking larger than they are. It is gain dependent and lowering the gain can decrease this. When lowering the gain weak doppler signals can be lost so doppler gain should be set by random noise. Aliasing is a doppler artefact when velocities of red blood cells are higher than the PRF. This occurs in areas of stenosis where reduced lumen of vessel is seen with a red to blue shift. Red represents flow towards the transducer and blue beyond the range of the PRF not reversed flow. Colour doppler artefacts are described further in the chapter 'Ultrasound in Large Vessel Vasculitis' [6, 7].

Common Ultrasound Features in Rheumatic Diseases?

When performing ultrasound and interpreting images, a structure will appear as being either anechoic, hypoechoic or hyperechoic relative to the surrounding tissue (Fig. 13) [2].

The synovium is usually hypoechoic within a joint, and any synovial fluid/effusion is described as being anechoic. Synovial fluid tends to be displaceable and

Fig. 13 Common features of structures seen on ultrasound i.e. black is anechoic usually relating to fluid, synovium is grey and hypoechoic

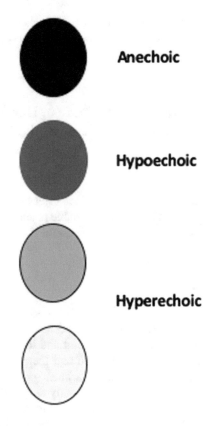

compressible and does not show any doppler signal. Synovial fluid may exhibit acoustic enhancement, demonstrated, by brighter echoes below. There is no doppler signal in healthy persons although very sensitive equipment may show minor flows in some joints [2].

Cartilage appears as a hypoechoic band over the bone and the bone appears as being a white hyperechoic structure [2].

Tendons and ligaments have a fine fibrillar pattern and are described as being hyperechoic if localised parallel to the probe. However, anisotropy can result if it is not parallel and the tendon may become hypoechoic or anechoic and simulate disease. This can be corrected by tilting the probe. Bursae are either hypoechoic or anechoic and commonly subacromial-subdeltoid bursa when examining the shoulder joint. Fibrocartilage such as the triangular fibrocartilage at the wrists, knee menisci and labrum in shoulders and hips can appear to be hyperechoic [2].

Nerves are hypoechoic, and their structure being dotted and less fibrillar. Median nerve on transverse view in carpal tunnel is sometimes described as being like a bunch of grapes or olives!!! [2]. Vessels are usually anechoic and colour and power doppler will demonstrate blood flow. This is the principle for use in scanning of temporal and axillary arteries in large vessel vasculitis (described later in the book).

The ultrasound practitioner should also be aware that subcutaneous adipose tissue can be either hypoechoic/midechoic and irregular. Muscles are generally hypoechoic but can be mid or hyperechoic [2].

A Step by Step Guide to Handling the Machine and the Probe and Approaching the Patent

Equipment

Large stationary machines offer a higher image quality and an improved range of functions. However, portable machines are able to offer similar resolutions and are more mobile and can be useful if scanning at the bedside/ward setting (Fig. 14).

Patient

A consideration should be made to the joint being examined and whether it is a superficial or deep joint and the patient's body habitus. Based on this the correct probe can be used and the patient seated appropriately. For example, for a shoulder examination a linear probe will be selected, and the patient placed on an examination chair usually at eye level of examiner. In contrast, to examine the feet the patient will be asked to sit on an examination couch and bend their knees and place their feet flat on the couch. The smaller joint can be seen better with a hockey stick probe (Fig. 15). It is important that the ultrasound practitioner is seated appropriately and preferably on a chair that swivels and comfortably to both see the ultrasound monitor and perform the examination.

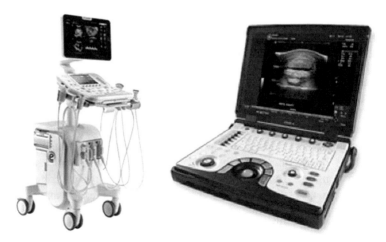

Fig. 14 Stationary versus portable machine

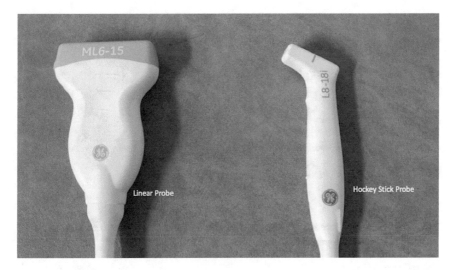

Fig. 15 Standard probes used in rheumatology ultrasound

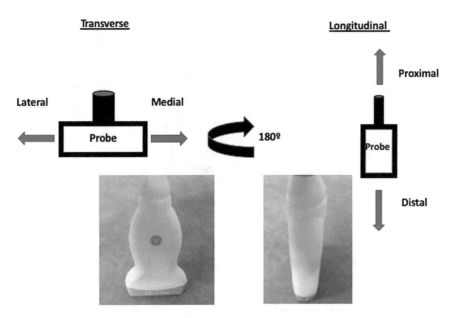

Fig. 16 Probe position in transverse followed by a 180 degree swivel and then in long axis

The Probe

There are several techniques that are employed when performing ultrasound examinations. The subject can be seen in a transverse or cross-sectional view and then by a 180° swivel on its axis the long axis or longitudinal view is obtained (Fig. 16). This can also be referred to as spinning. When in transverse the probe

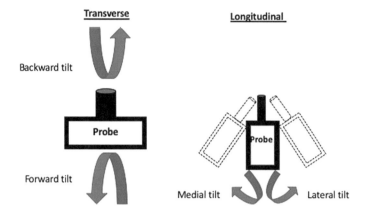

Fig. 17 Tilting of the probe in transverse (back and forwards) and then (side to side) in longitudinal

Fig. 18 Heel to toe manoeuvring to correct anisotropy in longitudinal plane especially when examining the biceps tendon

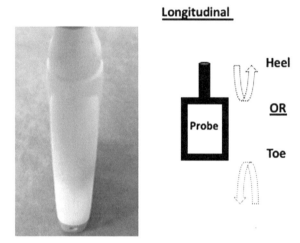

can be tilted backwards and forwards to correct any anisotropy . In longitudinal view the probe can tilted from side to side (Fig. 17). Heel- toe manoeuvre enables one part of the probe to be fixed at one end to a structure whilst the other end moves (Fig. 18). This is useful to avoid anisotropy especially when examining the biceps tendon in the bicipital groove [1, 2].

When handling the probe, we suggest using 3 fingers to hold then pen, very much like a pen, and use the remaining 2 (ulnar side) fingers to rest on the patient when examining. This will ensure that you are not exerting extra pressure on the structure being examined with the probe which can obscure findings (Figs. 19 and 20).

Fig. 19 Ideal probe position in transverse plane

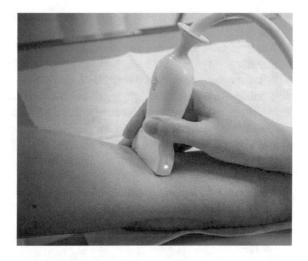

Fig. 20 Ideal probe position in longitudinal view

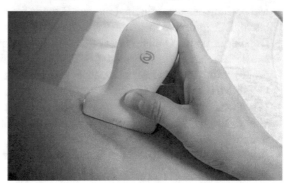

Probe/ Machine Setting

So once the correct probe has been selected and the patient is in the correct position for examination the following steps should be considered [8, 9]:

- Use left hand to adjust the machine controls and the right hand to examine the patient.
- Adjust the depth appropriate for the joint. A superficial joint will require a lower depth whereas a deeper joint will require a higher depth .
- The focus should be set at the point of interest. Some of the newer machines will do this automatically.
- The frequency should be adjusted according to the joint being examined. The superficial joints will require a high frequency and a lower frequency for deeper joint. Usually, this is done as part of a MSk preset and may not need to be done manually.
- The gain measures the power of sound waves. This is usually set on the machine settings.

- The freeze button is useful to pause an examination and review an image. It allows the operator a break from scanning.
- Power doppler/colour doppler should be identified and used appropriately.
- Measurement via the callipers is sometimes necessary.
- When machine settings are optimised, you are ready to scan. Ensure that when handling the probe, you don't apply too much pressure.
- Structures should be examined in both longitudinal (long axis) and transverse (short axis). When examining the same structure in 2 planes, a 180-degree swivel of the probe should be done on itself (Figs. 19 and 20).
- Any pathology seen should be confirmed in 2 planes (longitudinal and transverse).
- Images may be stored according to local protocol in your institution.

In 2017, EULAR [8, 9] published standardised procedures [10] to consider for those scanning and includes the following (some of which has been discussed in the chapter):

- MSUS includes two principal modes: B mode (or grey scale) that provides morphological information of the anatomic structures and Doppler mode (colour Doppler or power Doppler) that allows evaluation blood flow.
- MSUS should be performed with high resolution linear transducers i.e. probes with frequencies between 6 and 14 MHz for deep/intermediate areas to $\geq$15 MHz for superficial areas.
- When scanning a joint, the probe should be orientated as perpendicular or parallel to the bony cortical surface (bony acoustic landmark) so that the cortical margin appears bright, sharp and hyperechoic.
- A dynamic scanning technique by means of slight movements of transition (side to side, back to front) angulation and rotation of the probe should be carried out in order to allow best visualisation of the structures of interest.
- To avoid anisotropy (i.e. hypoechoic/anechoic appearance of a normally hyperechoic structure that mainly affects tendons), the probe should be continuously adjusted to maintain the beam perpendicular to the tendon fibres especially in insertional regions.
- When scanning in long axis, the most proximal aspect of the structure is usually placed on the left-hand side of the screen. Other options are acceptable as long as movement of the image on the screen is kept parallel to the direction of the probe on the patient.
- Probe compression can be helpful in distinguishing a compressible liquid collection from a non-compressible solid.
- Little or no compression is important when performing Doppler examination to avoid cessation of flow in small vessels.
- A generous amount of gel should be used for superficial structures especially when little or no pressure is indicated.
- The machine settings for B mode and Doppler mode should be optimised the US image acquisition process.

References

1. Iagnocco A, Naredo E, Bijlsma JWJ. Becoming a musculo-skeletal ultrasonographer. Best Pract Res Clin Rheumatol. 2013;27:271081.
2. Schmidt WA, Backhaus M. What the practising rheumatologist needs to know about the technical fundamentals of ultrasonography. Best Pract Res Clin Rheumatol. 2008;22(6):981–99.
3. Martinoli C. Gain setting in power Doppler. Radiology. 1997;202:284–85.
4. Kremkau FW. Doppler color imaging. Principles and Instrumentation. Clin Diagn Ultrasound. 1992;27:7–60.
5. Torp-Pedersen ST, Terslev L. Settings and artefacts relevant in colour/power doppler ultrasound in rheumatology. Ann Rheum Dis 2008;67:143–49.
6. Taljanovic MS, Melville DM, Scalcione LR, Gimber LH, Lorenz EJ, Witte RS. Artefacts in musculo-skeletal ultrasonography. Semin Musculoskeletal Radiol. 2014;18:3–11.
7. Terslev L, Diamantopolous AP, Dohn Moller U, Schmidt WA, Torp-Pedersen S. Setting and artefacts relevant for doppler ultrasound in large vessel vasculitis. Arthritis Res Ther. 2017;19:167.
8. Möller I, Janta I, Backhaus M, et al. The 2017 EULAR standardised procedures for ultrasound imaging in rheumatology. Ann Rheum Dis. 2017;76(12):1974–79.
9. Backhaus M, Burmester GR, Gerber T, Grassi W, Machold KP, Swen WA, et al. Guidelines for musculoskeletal ultrasound in rheumatology. Ann Rheum Dis. 2001;60:641–9.
10. Brown AK, O'connor PJ, Roberts TE, Wakefield RJ, Karim Z, Emery P. Recommendations for musculoskeletal ultrasonography by rheumatologists: setting global standards for best practice by expert consensus. Arthritis Rheum. 2005;53(1):83–92. https://doi.org/10.1002/art.20926.

The Wrist and Hand

Qasim Akram

Dorsal Examination of Wrist and Hand

Dorsal Wrist Examination

Basic Anatomy

The wrist joint is formed by the union of the distal radius and ulna with 8 carpal bones. It consists of the radio-ulnar joint, radio-carpal joint and mid carpal joints (Illustration 1) [1].

The 8 carpal bones are arranged in a proximal and a distal row. The proximal row includes Scaphoid, Lunate, Triquetrum and Pisiform. The distal row includes Trapezium, Trapezoid, Capitate and Hamate (Illustration 1). The carpal tunnel is formed by these bones and by a transverse carpal ligament called the flexor retinaculum (Illustrations 2 and 3). The triangular fibrocartilage is a biconcave disk positioned between the ulnar styloid and the trapezium (Illustration 4) [2].

There are 9 extensor tendons that are responsible for extension finger movements and run along the dorsal aspect (Illustration 5). There are 9 flexor tendons and these run along its volar aspect and are responsible for flexion movements of the fingers (Illustrations 2 and 3). The two wrist flexors, flexor carpi radialis and flexor carpi ulnaris, attach to the carpal bones and the palmaris longus tendon attaches to the transverse carpal ligament (flexor retinaculum) and palmar aponeurosis (Illustration 3) [1–3].

Lister's tubercle (of the radius) acts as a very useful landmark for US identification and is found between the 2nd and 3rd compartments [3, 4]. The first compartment, most radial, contains the abductor pollicis longus (APL) and extensor

Q. Akram (✉)
Stockport NHS Foundation Trust, Stockport, Greater Manchester, UK
e-mail: qasim.akram.qa@gmail.com

17

Illustration 1 Anatomical
illustration of the dorsal wrist
joint. Figure commissioned
by Dr Akram and printed
with permission from Unzag
Designs

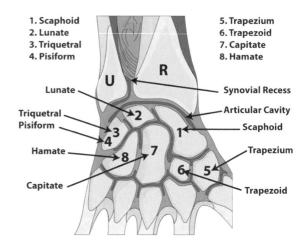

1. Scaphoid
2. Lunate
3. Triquetral
4. Pisiform

5. Trapezium
6. Trapezoid
7. Capitate
8. Hamate

Lunate — Synovial Recess
Triquetral — Articular Cavity
Pisiform — Scaphoid
Hamate — Trapezium
Capitate — Trapezoid

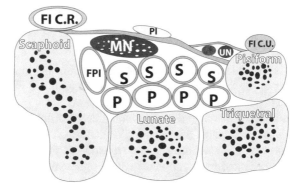

Illustration 2 Anatomical illustration of volar wrist and carpal tunnel- FLCR is flexor carpi radialis, Pl is palmarus longus, FLCU is flexor carpi ulnaris, MN is median nerve and UN is ulnar nerve. S is superficialis flexor tendons and P is profundus flexor tendons. FPI is flexor pollicis indicis. Figure commissioned by Dr Akram and printed with permission from Unzag Designs

pollicis brevis (EPB) tendons. Medial to this is the second extensor tendon compartment containing extensor carpi radialis longus (ECRL) and brevis (ECRB) which inserts on the base of the 2nd and 3rd metacarpals. The third compartment contains the extensor pollicis longus (EPL) tendon and is separated from the second one by Lister's tubercle. The 4th compartment is large and houses tendons of the extensor digitorum (EDC) and extensor indicis proprius (EIP) and includes the 2nd to 5th fingers. The 5th compartment encloses the extensor digiti minimi (EDM) and the 6th, most ulnar, includes extensor carpi ulnaris (ECU) which runs along distal ulna to insert on base of 5th metacarpal (Illustrations 5, 6, and 7) [4].

The main movements of the wrist and hand are flexion, extension, radial and ulna deviation as well as supination and pronation.

To begin the examination of the wrist and hand joint, the dorsal aspect of the wrist should be evaluated first. A linear probe is usually used for the wrist and

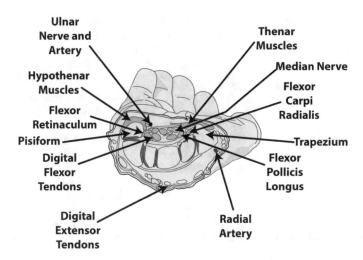

Illustration 3 Anatomical cross section illustration of carpal tunnel. Figure commissioned by Dr Akram and printed with permission from Unzag Designs

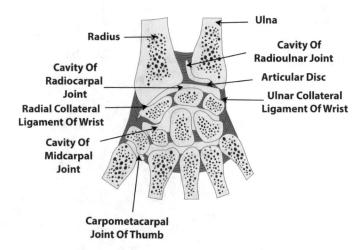

Illustration 4 Dorsal wrist joint including the articular disc on the ulnar aspect reflecting the triangular fibrocartilage. Figure commissioned by Dr Akram and printed with permission from Unzag Designs

hands (10–15 MHz) but a higher frequency probe (such as hockey stick) can be used mainly for the smaller, peripheral joints including an evaluation of the hyaline cartilage, sagittal bands, A1-A5 pulleys and extensor tendons at the level of the MCPJs and PIPJs. Ensure that adequate depth and focus is used. One hand should be used to control the US machine and its settings and the other to scan the relevant joint area [4, 5].

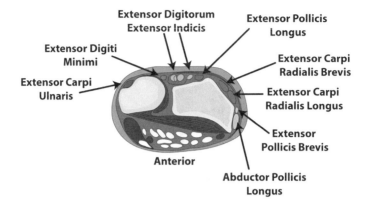

Illustration 5 Anatomical demonstration of the extensor tendons at the level of the wrist. Figure commissioned by Dr Akram and printed with permission from Unzag Designs

Illustration 6 Anatomical illustration of extensor tendons at the level of the wrist and also their insertion of the digits. Figure commissioned by Dr Akram and printed with permission from Unzag Designs

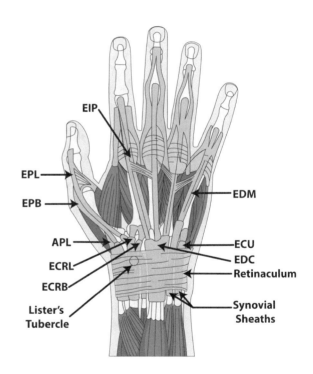

The patient is usually seated on a chair with hands resting on a flat surface in a prone position and in either neutral or a slight flexion (Fig. 1). Occasionally, a pillow can be used to support the hands. The examiner usually faces the patient.

The principal structures that can be evaluated on the dorsal wrist include the radio-ulnar joint, radio-carpal joint, carpo-metacarpal joints and the extensor tendon compartments (1–6).

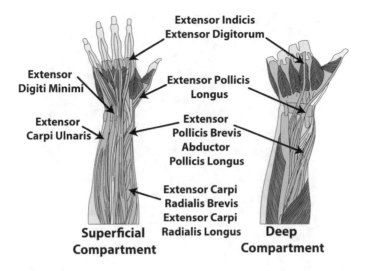

Illustration 7 Illustration of extensor tendons at wrist and digit level demonstrating superficial and deep compartments. Figure commissioned by Dr Akram and printed with permission from Unzag Designs

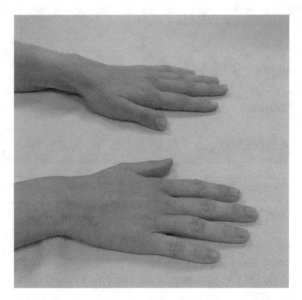

Fig. 1 Patient position and probe position (starting point) for the evaluation of the wrist joint

Radio-Ulnar Joint

The evaluation of the dorsal wrist starts off with a longitudinal view (Figs. 2 and 3) of the radio-ulnar joint. The forearm is in a prone position with flexion at the elbow joint and palms flat on the examination couch. The probe is positioned in longitudinal at the distal radius and ulna and then swept from proximal to distal.

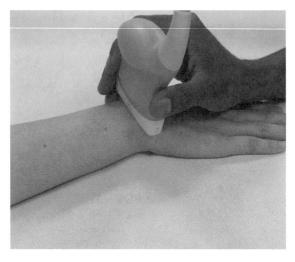

Fig. 2 Patient position and probe position (starting point) for the longitudinal evaluation of the radio-ulnar joint

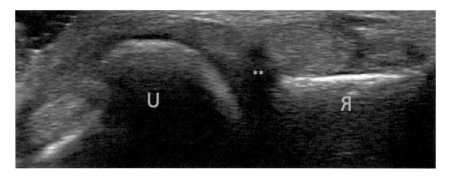

Fig. 3 Longitudinal view of the radio-ulnar joint. R = represents radius. U-represents ulna

Radio-Carpal and Mid-Carpal Joint

Remaining in the same position, the probe is moved to have a look at the radio-carpal joint in a longitudinal view in line with the 3rd metacarpal or 3rd finger. The probe is usually swept distally towards the carpo-metacarpal joint identifying the radius, lunate and capitate along the course of the probe (Figs. 4 and 5). The probe should be swept from proximal to distal and from medial to lateral [4, 5].

Extensor Tendons and Lister's Tubercle

Following this, an examination of the each of the individual extensor tendon compartments (1–6) should be made at the level of Lister's tubercle. The patient's position remains the same. The probe is placed at the level of Lister's tubercle

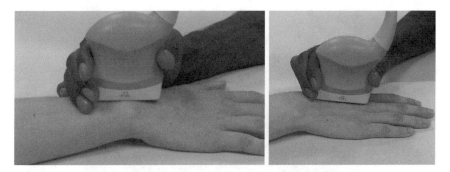

Fig. 4 Patient position and probe position for the longitudinal evaluation of the radio-carpal joint (4.1), mid-carpal joint and carpo-metacarpal joint (4.2). Probe is moved from proximal to distal to evaluate the radio-carpal joint, mid-carpal joints and then the carpo-metacarpal joint

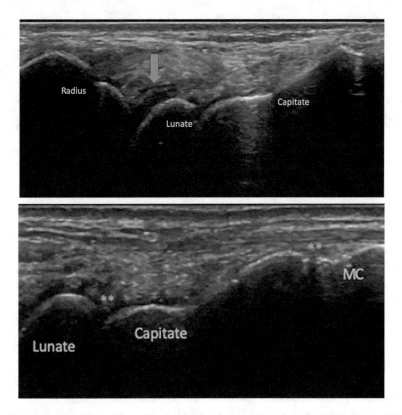

Fig. 5 Longitudinal view of the radio-carpal joint. Landmarks include Radius, Lunate and Capitate. Arrows point towards radio-carpal joint. 5.2-Mid-carpal joint and carpo-metacarpal joints. Landmarks: Lunate, Capitate, MC = metacarpal. ** carpo-metacarpal joint

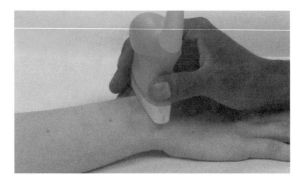

Fig. 6 Patient position and probe position of the transverse view of the extensor tendons

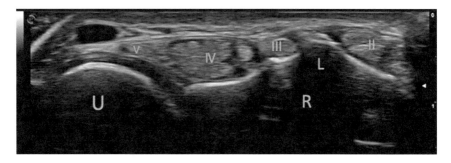

Fig. 7 Transverse view of extensor tendons. R = Radius, U = ulna, L = lister's tubercle. (II, III, IV, V) represents the 2nd, 3rd, 4th and 5th extensor tendon compartments at the level of the wrist joint

and the ulna styloid. The extensor retinaculum can also be assessed at this level (Figs. 6 and 7).

The 2nd extensor compartment is identified which compromises the ECRL, ECRB. These sit on the medial aspect of the Lister's tubercle on the lateral radius (Figs. 8 and 9) [2].

To examine the 1st extensor tendon compartment, the wrist is semi pronated, and the hand is placed halfway between supination and pronation position (Figs. 10 and 11). The probe is placed in transverse over the radial styloid. The probe is swept from medial to lateral to examine entire extensor tendon of APL and EPB in a transverse view. The probe is then placed in a longitudinal view (Figs. 12 and 13) and swept from proximal to distal. The radial styloid is identified, and the scaphoid tubercle can be seen if probe is swept distally [4].

The wrist is then placed back into the original position (elbow flexed, wrist pronated). The probe is then moved to the lateral aspect of the Lister's tubercle and the 3rd extensor tendon (EPL) is identified in the transverse view (Figs. 14 and 15).

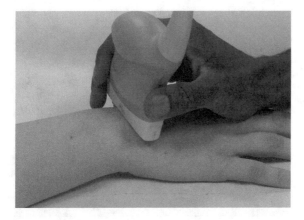

Fig. 8 Patient position and probe position transverse view of the 2nd extensor tendon compartment

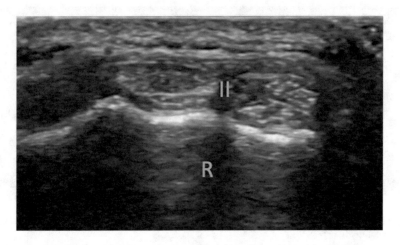

Fig. 9 Transverse scan of the 2nd extensor tendon compartment. (II) represents the 2nd extensor tendon compartment

Moving the probe more laterally the 4th extensor tendon (EDC, EIP) is seen and this compromises the extensor digits at the level of the radio-ulnar joint (Figs. 16 and 17).

The 5th extensor tendon (EDM) is seen on the medial aspect of the ulnar styloid (Figs. 18 and 19).

To examine the 6th extensor tendon (ECU) the wrist is placed in a slight radial deviation. The probe is placed in the ulnar groove in a transverse view and the 6th extensor tendon (ECU) is identified (Figs. 20 and 21). The probe is swept from medial to lateral. A longitudinal view of the 6th extensor tendon (ECU) is made, and the probe is swept from proximal to distal. The distal ulna and triquetrum

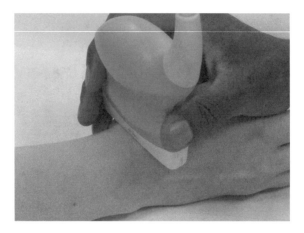

Fig. 10 Patient position and probe position transverse view of the 1st extensor tendon compartment

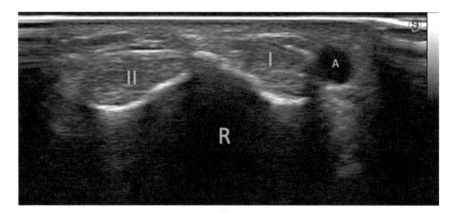

Fig. 11 Transverse scan of the 1st extensor tendon compartment. (I) represents the 1st extensor tendon compartment

are seen in the sonoanatomy image (Figs. 22 and 23). The triangular fibrocartilage (TFCC) can also be identified in this plane (Fig. 23). An important point is to reduce the frequency and increase gain for echogenicity such as identifying crystal deposition in the TFCC which occurs in pseudo-gout [4, 6].

Scapho-Lunate Ligament

The scapho-lunate ligament is then seen, in the same position but now with a hand placed in a slight flexion. The probe is placed in transverse between scaphoid and lunate. You should see 4th ET and scaphoid and lunate bones (Figs. 24 and 25) [4].

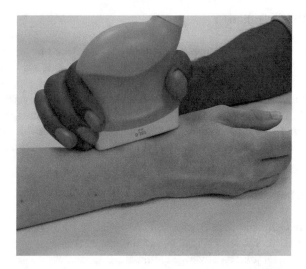

Fig. 12 Patient position and probe position longitudinal view of the 1st extensor tendon compartment

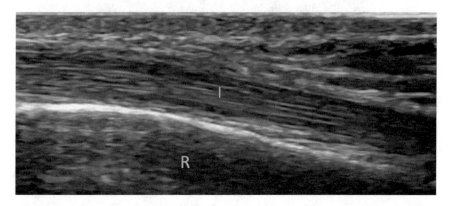

Fig. 13 Longitudinal scan of the 1st extensor tendon compartment. (I) represents the 1st extensor tendon compartment

Dorsal Thumb MCP and CMCJ (Illustration 8)

Then an examination of the small joints of the hand can be made. To start with, the 1st CMC is examined in a long axis view down to the thumb MCPJ. The hands should be placed in a semi prone position similar to the position for the 1st extensor tendon compartment (Figs. 26 and 27).

Dorsal MCP (Illustration 8)

The hand can be placed in either a neutral or slightly flexed position. An examination of the MCP joint is carried out initially in a long axis view (Figs. 28 and 29) followed by a transverse view (Figs. 30 and 31). The probe should be swept laterally and medially ensuring a look at the extensor tendon, synovial joint and hyaline cartilage in transverse view. The sagittal bands (illustration 9) can also be identified at this level. To examine the cartilage thoroughly a full flexion of the MCP should be made. The easiest way is to ask the patient to make a fist [4, 5].

Dorsal PIP (Illustration 8)

The probe can be moved distally to identify the PIPJ in both longitudinal (Figs. 32 and 33) and transverse views (Figs. 34 and 35) ensuring a close look at the extensor tendon, synovial joint and hyaline cartilage.

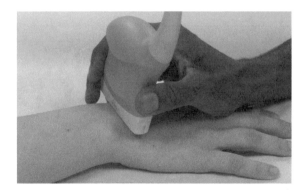

Fig. 14 Patient position and probe position transverse view of the 3rd extensor tendon compartment

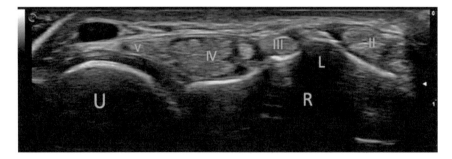

Fig. 15 Transverse scan of the 3rd[t] extensor tendon compartment. (III) represents the 3rd extensor tendon compartment

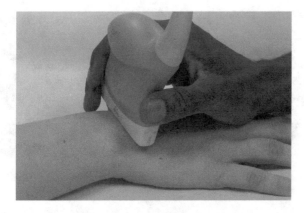

Fig. 16 Patient position and probe position transverse view of the 4th extensor tendon compartment

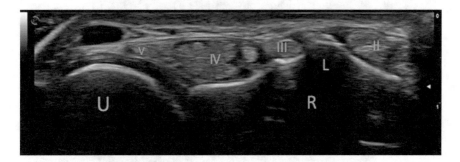

Fig. 17 Transverse scan of the 4th extensor tendon compartment. (IV) represents the 4th extensor tendon compartment

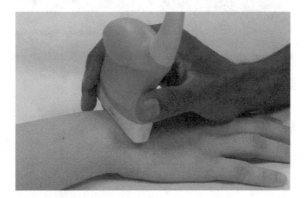

Fig. 18 Patient position and probe position transverse view of the 5th extensor tendon compartment

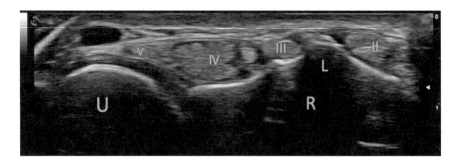

Fig. 19 Transverse scan of the 5th extensor tendon compartment. (V) represents the 5th extensor tendon compartment

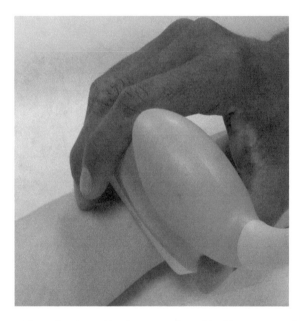

Fig. 20 Patient position and probe position transverse view of the 6th extensor tendon compartment

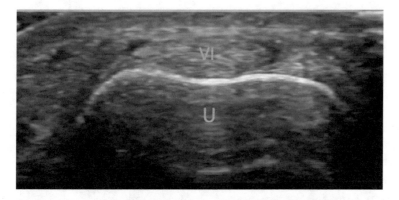

Fig. 21 Transverse scan of the 6th extensor tendon compartment. Landmarks-VI. U = Ulna. (VI) represents the 6th extensor tendon compartment

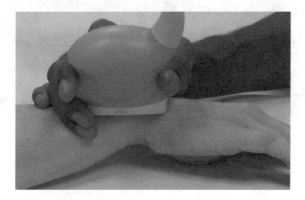

Fig. 22 Patient position and probe position longitudinal view of the 6th extensor tendon compartment

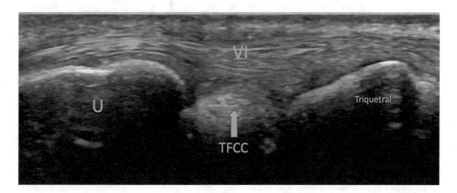

Fig. 23 Longitudinal scan of the 6th extensor tendon compartment. (VI) represents the 6th extensor tendon compartment. TFCC = Triangular fibrocartilage. Triquetral bone

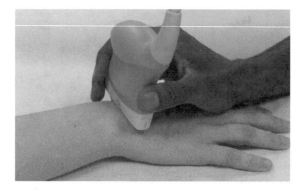

Fig. 24 Patient position and probe position transverse view of the scapho-lunate ligament

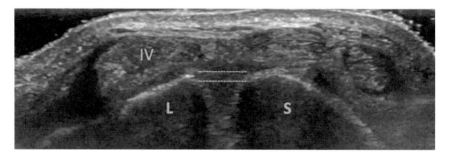

Fig. 25 Transverse scan of the scapho-lunate ligament. Landmarks-Lunate, Scaphoid and dashed lines is SL ligament. (IV) represents the 4th compartment

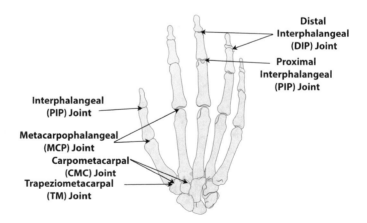

Illustration 8 Anatomical illustration of the small joints of the hand including the CMCJ and thumb MCPJ as well as other MCPJs, PIPJs, and DIPJs. Figure commissioned by Dr Akram and printed with permission from Unzag Designs

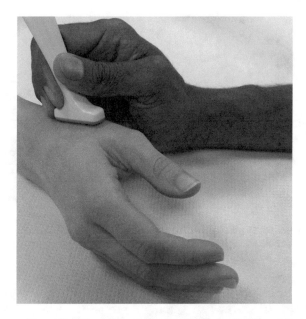

Fig. 26 Patient position and probe position for the longitudinal evaluation of the 1st CMC joint

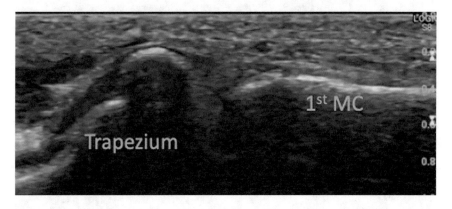

Fig. 27 Longitudinal scan of the 1st CMC joint. Landmarks-trapezium and 1st MC-metacarpal

Dorsal DIP (Illustration 8)

The probe is moved further distal to examine the DIPJ and again looking at the synovial joint, underlying bone and extensor tendon (Figs. 36 and 37).

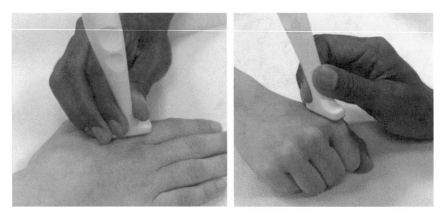

Fig. 28 Patient and probe position for the longitudinal evaluation of the dorsal MCPJ (28.1). Flexion demonstrates better view of the MCP joint cartilage (28.1)

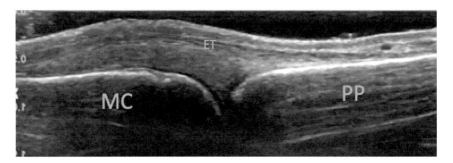

Fig. 29 Longitudinal evaluation of the dorsal MCPJ. Landmarks = MC-metacarpal, PP-proximal phalanx. ET-extensor tendon. MCPJ represents the joint capsule

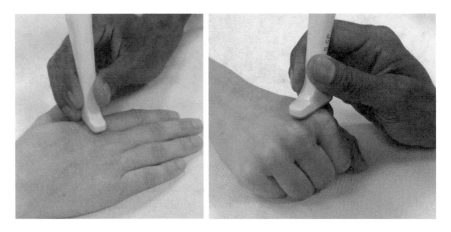

Fig. 30 Patient and probe position for the transverse evaluation of the dorsal MCPJ (30.1) and in flexion (30.2)

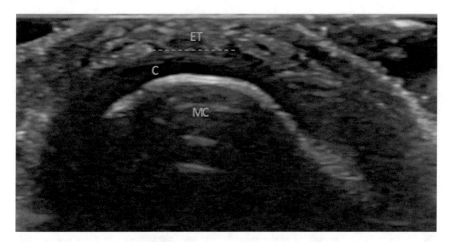

Fig. 31 Transverse evaluation of the dorsal MCPJ. MC-metacarpal, C-cartilage, ET-extensor tendon. Dotted line represents sagittal band

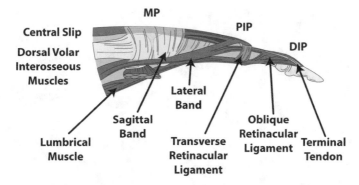

Illustration 9 Anatomical illustration of dorsal MCP(MP), PIP and DIP. Figure commissioned by Dr Akram and printed with permission from Unzag Designs

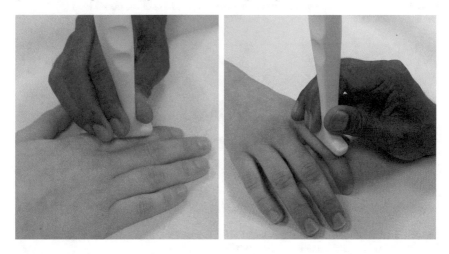

Fig. 32 Patient and probe position for the longitudinal evaluation of the dorsal PIPJ and in flexion (32.1)

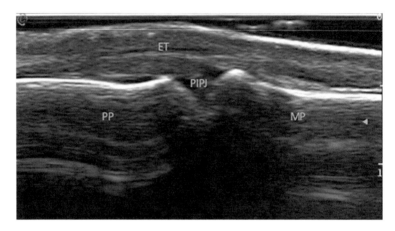

Fig. 33 Longitudinal evaluation of the dorsal PIPJ. Landmarks-PP-proximal phalanx, MP-middle phalanx. ET-extensor tendon. PIPJ represents the joint capsule

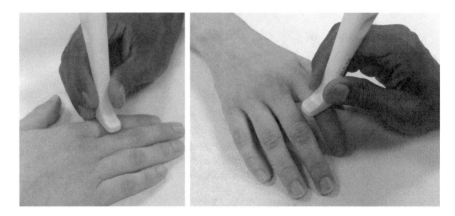

Fig. 34 Patient and probe position for the transverse evaluation of the dorsal PIPJ (34.1) and in full flexion (34.2)

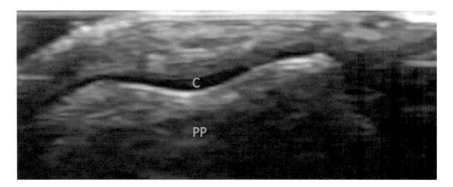

Fig. 35 Transverse evaluation of the dorsal PIPJ. Ensure look at ET-extensor tendon, synovial joint and C-hyaline cartilage. PP-proximal phalanx

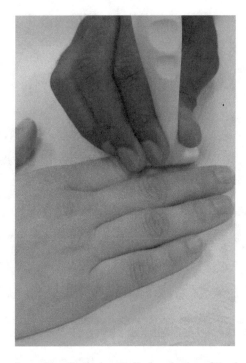

Fig. 36 Patient and probe position for the longitudinal evaluation of the dorsal DIPJ

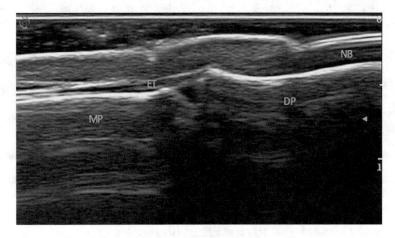

Fig. 37 Longitudinal evaluation of the dorsal DIPJ. MP-middle phalanx. DP-distal phalanx. ET-extensor tendon. NP-nail plate. DIPJ represent the joint capsule

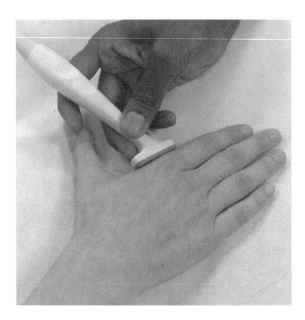

Fig. 38 Patient and probe position for the evaluation of the MCPJ radial collateral ligament. This can be done for PIPJs and DIPJs with similar principles

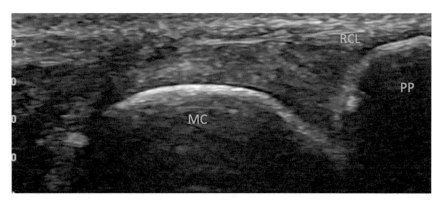

Fig. 39 Longitudinal evaluation of the MCPJ radial collateral bands. Landmarks-MC-metacarpal. PP-proximal phalanx. RCL is radial collateral ligament

Collateral Ligaments (MCPJs and PIPJs) (Illustration 9)

To look at the collateral ligament of the MCPJ, the probe is positioned between MC heads and proximal phalanges and probe is swept in long axis. You should see MC heads, proximal phalanges and volar plate. The collateral ligament should be seen in both radial (RCL) and ulna (UCL) views (Figs. 38, 39, 40, and 41) [4].

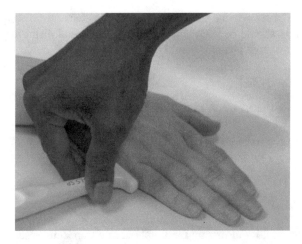

Fig. 40 Patient and probe position for the evaluation of the MCPJ ulna collateral ligaments. This can be done for PIPJs and DIPJs with similar principles

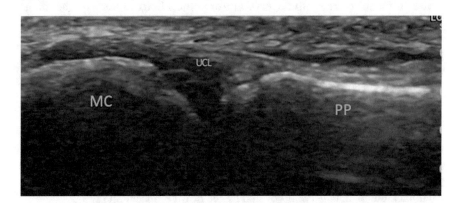

Fig. 41 Longitudinal evaluation of the MCPJ ulna collateral ligaments. Landmarks-MC-metacarpal. PP-proximal phalanx. UCL is ulna collateral ligament

For the collateral ligaments of the PIPJ, the probe is placed between proximal and middle phalanges. This should be repeated on both radial (RCL) and ulna (UCL) views. Proximal phalanges, ligament and the middle phalanges should be seen.

Thumb Collateral Ligament (Illustration 9)

In terms of the thumb ulnar collateral ligament the forearm should be in a semi prone position with abduction of the thumb. The elbow is flexed of course. The probe is placed between the MC and proximal phalanx. Both longitudinal and transverse views should be seen and medial to lateral and distal to proximal. 1st MC head and proximal phalanx should be seen.

Volar Examination of Wrist and Hand

Volar Wrist (Radio-Carpal Joint, Carpal Tunnel, Median Nerve, Flexor Tendons)

Basic Anatomy (Illustrations 2 and 3)

The flexor retinaculum inserts on the scaphoid and trapezium (radial side) and on the pisiform and hook of hamate (ulnar side) to form the carpal tunnel [1–3].

The 9 flexor tendons traverse the carpal tunnel and reach the fingers. 4 tendons are from the flexor digitorum superficialis (2nd to 5th fingers) and 4 flexor digitorum profundus (2nd to 5th fingers). Flexor pollicis longus inserts on the thumb. The wrist flexors, flexor carpi radialis (FCR) and flexor carpi ulnaris (FCU), lie outside the carpal tunnel and are more superficial. The FCR tendon inserts on palmar aspect of base of 2nd metacarpal and allows flexion and radial deviation of wrist. The FCU courses on ulnar side of wrist housing pisiform and inserts on hook of hamate and 5th MCP. This allows flexion and ulnar deviation of the wrist. The palmaris longus is thin and absent in 20% of individuals. It tends to cross the midline and is superficial to the flexor retinaculum [1, 2].

Inside the carpal tunnel, the median nerve runs superficial to the tendons of flexor pollicis longus and flexor digitorum superficialis tendons. The nerve has on oval cross section at the proximal tunnel and tends to become more flattened as it progresses distally through the tunnel (level of the hamate hook). Through the carpal tunnel, the median nerve is covered by the flexor retinaculum [2, 3].

So, following the completed examination of the dorsal wrist and hand, the wrist is then turned over to a supine position and in a minimal flexion position at the wrists resting on the examination couch (or a flat surface). The elbow is still being maintained in a flexion. At this position, the probe is placed in a long axis view over the volar wrist identifying the superficial median nerve, and radio-carpal bones inferior to this. The probe is swept from proximal and distal (Figs. 42, 43, and 44).

The probe is then swivelled 180 degrees in transverse view to identify the carpal tunnel including the median nerve and the flexor tendons. The probe is placed between the scaphoid tubercle and pisiform over the flexor retinaculum. On the sonoanatomy image you should see the scaphoid, pisiform proximally and moving the probe distally the trapezium and hook of hamate should be seen (Figs. 45 and 46) [4].

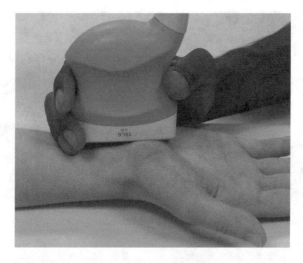

Fig. 42 Patient position and probe position for the longitudinal evaluation of the dorsal wrist joint and median nerve

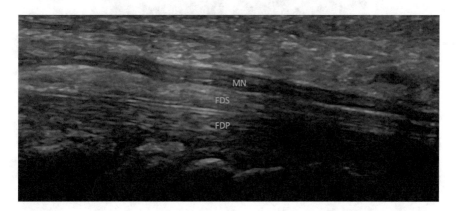

Fig. 43 Longitudinal scan of the median nerve. Landmarks-MN-median nerve. FDS-Flexor digitorum superficialis

Flexor Tendons of Wrist (and FPL)

Basic Anatomy

The flexor digitorum superficialis (SFD or FDS) and flexor digitorum profundus (PFD or FDP) act together to flex the MCP and PIPJ. The PFD or FDP acts on the distal phalanx to create flexion (Illustrations 10 and 11) [3, 4].

The annular pulleys are located at five specific points along the tendon sheath and are numbered proximal to distal.

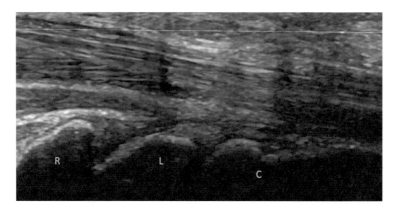

Fig. 44 Longitudinal scan of the radio-carpal joint. R = radius, L = Lunate and C = capitate

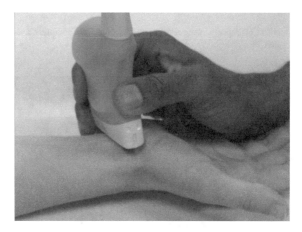

Fig. 45 Patient position and probe position for the transverse evaluation of the carpal tunnel

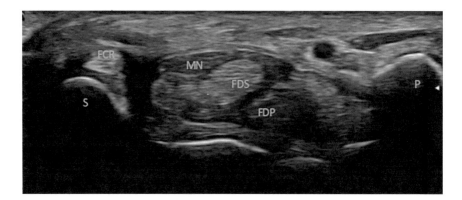

Fig. 46 Transverse scan of the carpal tunnel and median nerve. Note the S-scaphoid, P-pisiform proximally and trapezium and hamate distally. FCR-flexor carpi radialis, MN-median nerve, FDS-flexor digitorum superficialis, FDP-flexor digitorum profundus

The first A1 extends from area of palmar plate of MCPJ to base of proximal phalanx, the second (A2) extends from base of proximal phalanx to junction of the proximal two thirds and the distal third of the proximal phalanx. A3 is small in size and located over PIPJ, A4 is in middle third of middle phalanx and A5 is in distal interphalangeal joint (Illustration 12) [2, 3].

Keeping the same position, the probe is placed transverse over flexor retinaculum between scaphoid tubercle and pisiform. The probe is swept from medial to lateral (Figs. 45 and 46) identifying the flexor tendons at the level of the wrist [4].

The probe is then moved down to the thumb to identify the FPL tendon in both long axis and transverse views (Figs. 47, 48, 49, and 50).

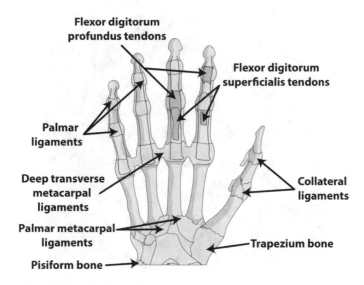

Illustration 10 Anatomical illustration of the flexor tendons and ligaments of the small joints. Figure commissioned by Dr Akram and printed with permission from Unzag Designs

Illustration 11 Anatomical illustration of digital flexor tendons. In (a) level of the MCPJ (MC), in (b) level of proximal phalanx (PP), in (c) level of middle phalanx (MP). SFD is superficialis flexor tendon and PFD is profundus flexor digitorum. Figure commissioned by Dr Akram and printed with permission from Unzag Designs

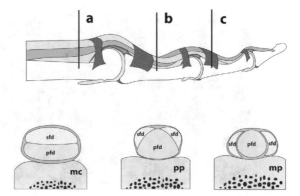

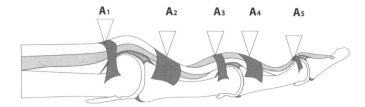

Illustration 12 Illustration of the flexor tendon pulleys- A1 is at the level of MCPJ, A2/A3 at the proximal phalanx and A4/A5 at the middle phalanx. Figure commissioned by Dr Akram and printed with permission from Unzag Designs

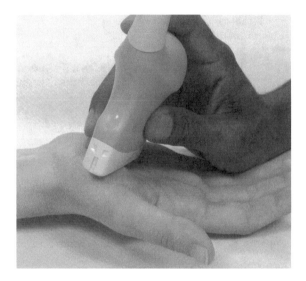

Fig. 47 Patient position and probe position for the transverse evaluation of the flexor pollicis longus

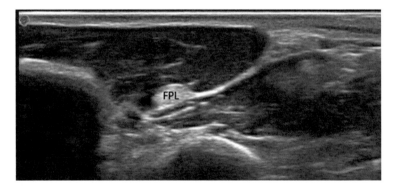

Fig. 48 Transverse scan of the flexor pollicis longus tendon. Landmarks is FPL-flexor pollicis longus tendon

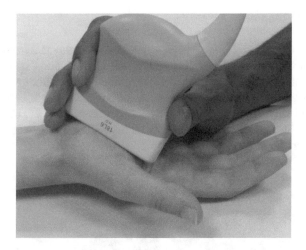

Fig. 49 Patient position and probe position for the longitudinal evaluation of the flexor pollicis longus

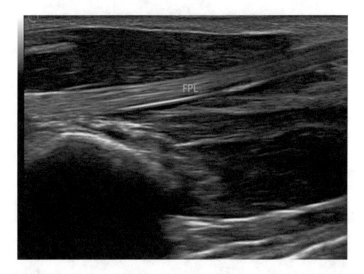

Fig. 50 Longitudinal scan of the flexor pollicis longus tendon. Landmark is FPL-flexor pollicis longus tendon

Volar 1st CMCJ

The thumb can then be extended. A long axis view is obtained by placing the probe on the base of 1st or thumb MC bone and trapezium of the carpus. The probe is swept from distal to proximal (Figs. 51 and 52).

Finger Flexor Tendons

The probe is then placed in a transverse position over the MC heads to identify the finger flexor tendons. Then each individual flexor tendon is examined in a longitudinal and then a transverse view. The probe is swept from proximal to distal in long axis and medial to lateral in transverse view. The MC bone and phalanges should be seen (Figs. 53, 54, 55, 56, 57, 58, 59, 60, 61, 62, 63, and 64) (Illustration 12). The FDS or SFD inserts on the middle phalanx, and the FDP or PFD inserts on the distal phalanx [3, 4].

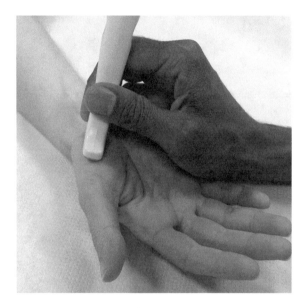

Fig. 51 Patient position and probe position for the longitudinal evaluation of the volar 1st CMCJ

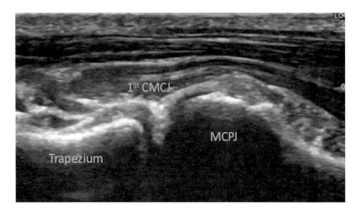

Fig. 52 Longitudinal view of the 1st CMCJ. Landmarks-Tr-trapezium, CMCJ, MCPJ

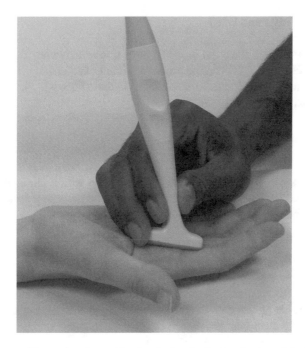

Fig. 53 Patient position and probe position for the longitudinal evaluation of the flexor tendons at the MCPJs as well as the MCPJ

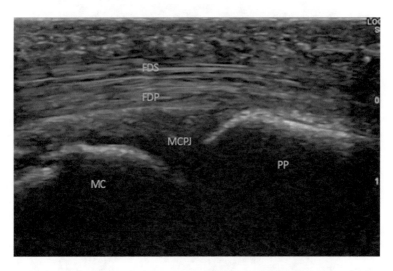

Fig. 54 Longitudinal scan of the flexor tendons at the MCPJs. MC-metacarpal, PP-proximal phalanx, MCPJ. FDS-flexor digitorum superficialis and FDP-flexor digitorum profundus

Volar MCPJ, PIPJ and DIPJ

In the same position, place the probe to have a long axis view of MCP (including thumb), PIP, DIPJs. Sweep the probe proximally and distally. Transverse view should be obtained sweeping from medial to lateral (Figs. 53, 54, 55, 56, 57, 58, 59, 60, 61, 62, 63, and 64) [4, 5].

Pulleys

A1-A5 pulleys can also be seen in the same position with a minimal dorsiflexion of the wrist and minimal extension of the fingers. The probe is placed in longitudinal over MC heads and phalanges (Figs. 65 and 66) [4, 5].

Pathology

The reason for using ultrasound in rheumatology is to detect abnormal pathology which can enable an accurate diagnosis especially at the point of care. The wrist and hand are the most frequent sites to be involved in rheumatological disease [7].

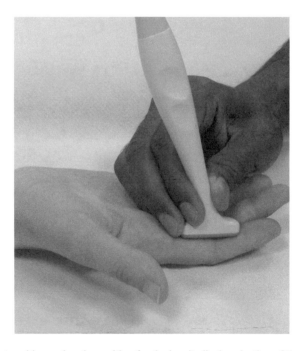

Fig. 55 Patient position and probe position for the longitudinal evaluation of the flexor tendons at the PIPJs as well as the PIPJ

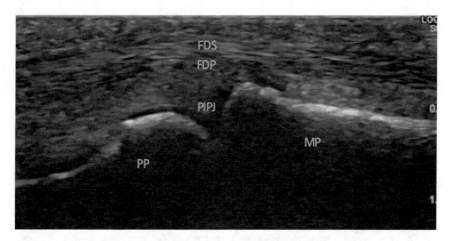

Fig. 56 Longitudinal scan of the flexor tendons at the PIPJs., PP-proximal phalanx, MP-middle phalanx. FDS-flexor digitorum superficialis and FDP-flexor digitorum profundus. Note-FDS inserts onto middle phalanx and FDP continues onto distal phalanx

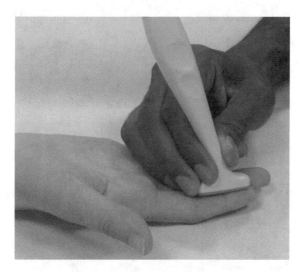

Fig. 57 Patient position and probe position for the longitudinal evaluation of the flexor tendons at the DIPJs as well as the DIPJs

The evaluation of the radio-ulnar, radio-carpal and midcarpal joints as well as the MCPJ, PIPJs and DIPJs can detect effusion or synovitis/synovial hypertrophy. This may also have a positive power doppler signal (Figs. 67, 68, 69, 70, 71, and 72). Erosions can be seen (Fig. 73). This is usually present in inflammatory arthritis such as rheumatoid arthritis, spondyloarthropathy, crystal arthritis, inflammatory osteoarthritis and septic arthritis [6].

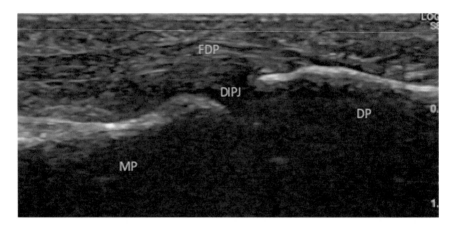

Fig. 58 Longitudinal scan of the flexor tendons at the DIPJs. MP-middle phalanx, DP-distal phalanx. DIPJ-joint. FDP-flexor digitorum profundus

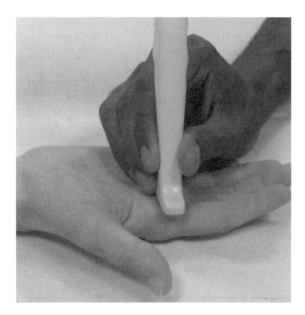

Fig. 59 Patient position and probe position for the transverse evaluation of the flexor tendons at the level of MCPJs

An assessment of these joints can also indicate osteoarthritis. Osteoarthritis causes characteristic osteophytes which can be seen at the DIPJ (Fig. 74), PIPJs and MCPJs. Spondyloarthopathies such as Psoriatic arthritis can affect the DIPJs whereas Rheumatoid arthritis will only affect as far up to the PIPJs. Although, beyond the scope of this book nail involvement can also be seen in psoriatic arthritis on ultrasound [6].

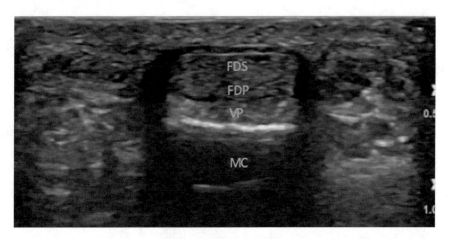

Fig. 60 Transverse scan of the flexor tendons at the MCPJs. FDS-flexor digitorum superficialis and FDP-flexor digitorum profundus. VP-volar plate

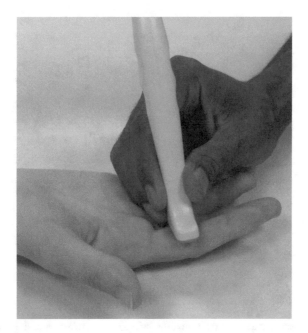

Fig. 61 Patient position and probe position for the transverse evaluation of the flexor tendons at the level of proximal phalanx

An assessment of the tendons at both wrist and digit level (including the extensor tendon compartments and flexor tendons) and ligaments can detect tenosynovitis, enthesopathy or tears. This is usually caused by spondyloarthropathy or rheumatoid arthritis. Mechanical overuse or trauma may cause tendon or ligament tears. Tendon and ligament tears may be observed as an anechoic or hypoechoic

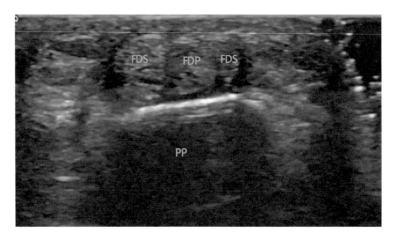

Fig. 62 Transverse scan of the flexor tendons at the proximal phalanx. FDS-flexor digitorum superficialis and FDP-flexor digitorum profundus. VP-volar plate

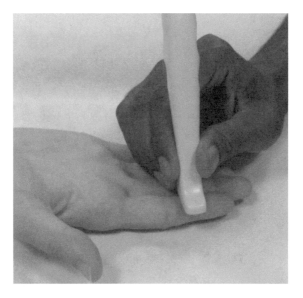

Fig. 63 Patient position and probe position for the transverse evaluation of the flexor tendons at the level of middle phalanx

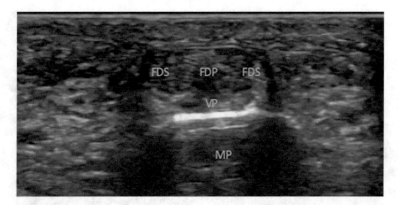

Fig. 64 Transverse scan of the flexor tendons at the middle phalanx. FDS-flexor digitorum superficialis and FDP-flexor digitorum profundus. VP-volar plate. Note-this is where FDS terminates onto the middle phalanx

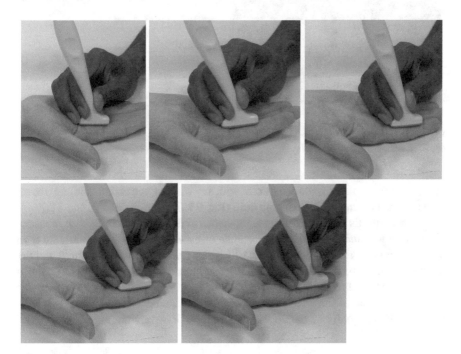

Fig. 65 Patient position and probe position for the longitudinal evaluation of the flexor pulleys-65.1-A1, 65.2-A2, 65.3-A3, 65.4-A4, 65.5-A5

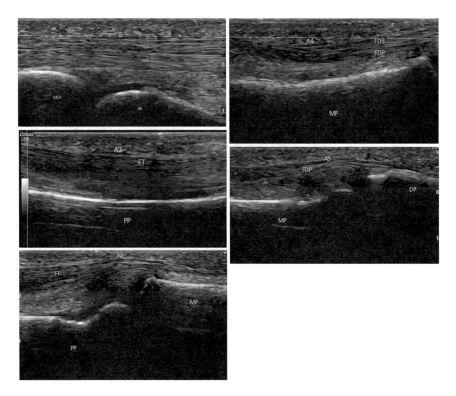

Fig. 66 Longitudinal scan of the individual flexor tendon pulleys-66.1-A1, 66.2-A2, 66.3-A3, 66.4-A4, 66.5-A5

discontinuity of the fibrillary pattern with or without retraction and, in recent cases, with surrounding hypoechoic fluid (Fig. 75, 76, 77, 78, 79, 80, and 81).

Crystal arthritis commonly affects the hands and wrists including both monosodium urate goutand calcium pyrophosphate disease. These can commonly be seen at sites including the triangular fibrocartilage as a bright hyperechoic area and the hyaline cartilage of the MCPJs as a double contour sign (Fig. 82). Tophi can also be seen at the level of the interphalangeal joints.

An assessment of the median nerve can demonstrate common pathologies such as carpal tunnel syndrome commonly caused by wrist synovitis (Figs. 83 and 84).

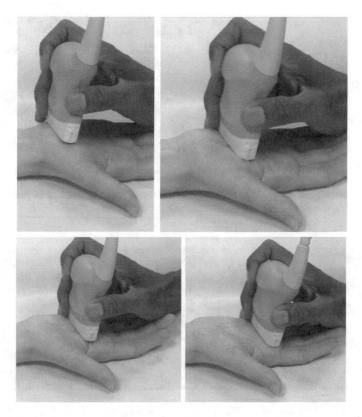

Fig. 67 Patient and probe position for a sweep of the flexor tendons of the palms

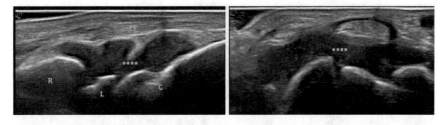

Fig. 68 Longitudinal scan of the radiocarpal joint demonstrating synovitis (***) in a patient with rheumatoid arthritis. R = Radius, L = Lunate, C = capitate

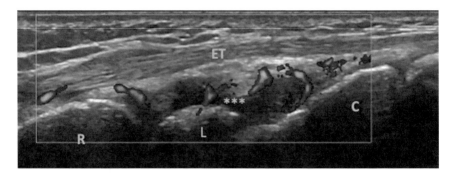

Fig. 69 Longitudinal scan of the radiocarpal joint demonstrating synovitis with power doppler activity (***). R = Radius, L = Lunate, C = capitate. Typical of rheumatoid arthritis

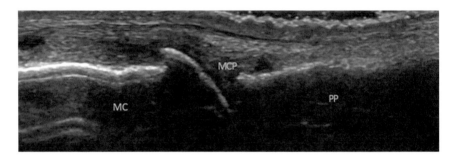

Fig. 70 Longitudinal scan of the MCPJ showing synovitis. Notice the dark around the MCPJ. Typical of rheumatoid arthritis but also seen in Psoriatic arthritis

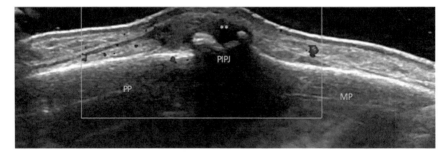

Fig. 71 Longitudinal scan of the PIPJ showing synovitis (**). PP-proximal phalanx. MP-middle phalanx. Typical of rheumatoid arthritis but also seen in Psoriatic arthritis

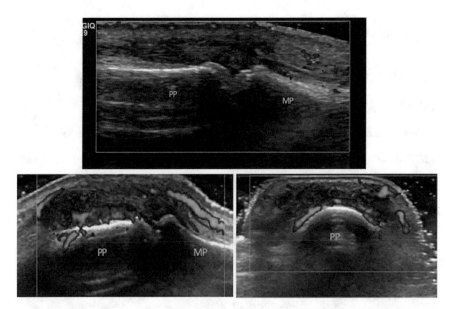

Fig. 72 1. Longitudinal scan of the PIPJ showing synovitis and doppler activity. 2. Transverse scan of PIPJ. PP-middle phalanx. Typical of rheumatoid arthritis but also seen in Psoriatic arthritis

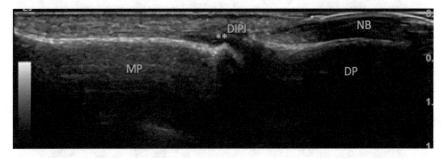

Fig. 73 Longitudinal scan of the DIPJ showing synovitis (**). PP-proximal phalanx. DP-distal phalanx. NB-nail bed. Typical of Psoriatic arthritis

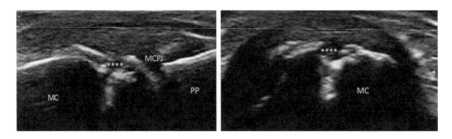

Fig. 74 A. Longitudinal scan of the MCPJ showing erosions and B. Transverse scan of MCPJ showing erosion (****). MC-metacarpal and PP-proximal phalanx

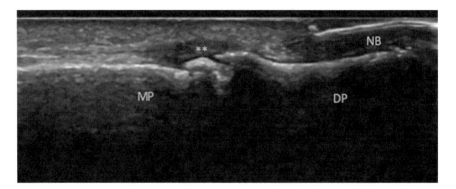

Fig. 75 Longitudinal scan of the DIPJ showing osteophytes and associated synovial hypertrophy (**). MP-middle phalanx and DP-distal phalanx. NB-nail bed. Typical of osteoarthritis

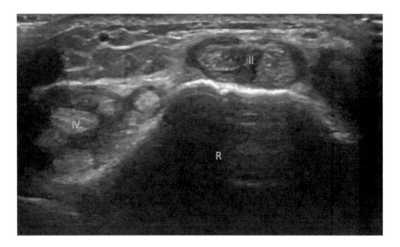

Fig. 76 Transverse scan of the 2nd (II), 3rd (III), 4th (IV) extensor tendons demonstrating tenosynovitis. R-Radius. Note: dark areas around the tendons

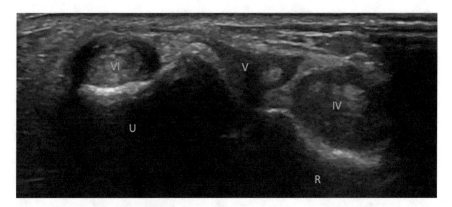

Fig. 77 Transverse scan of the 4th (IV), 5th (V), 6th (VI) extensor tendons demonstrating teno-synovitis. R-Radius. U-ulna. Note: dark areas around the tendons. Typical of rheumatoid arthritis but also seen in Psoriatic arthritis

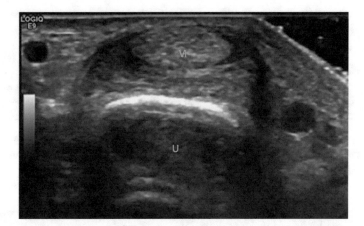

Fig. 78 Transverse scan of the 6th (VI) extensor tendon demonstrating tenosynovitis. U-ulna. Note: dark areas around the tendons. Typical of rheumatoid arthritis but also seen in Psoriatic arthritis

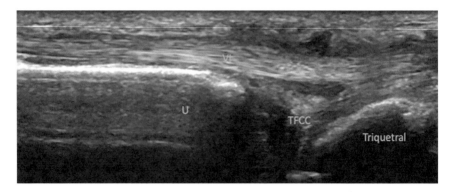

Fig. 79 Longitudinal scan of the 6th (VI) extensor tendon demonstrating tenosynovitis. U-ulna. TFCC-triangular fibrocartilage. Note: dark areas around the tendons. Typical of rheumatoid arthritis but also seen in Psoriatic arthritis

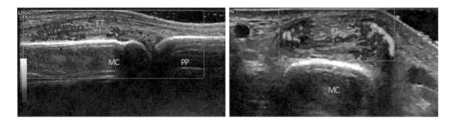

Fig. 80 **a** Longitudinal scan of the MCPJ showing (ET) extensor tendon with doppler activity and **b**. Transverse scan of MCPJ showing tenosynovitis of the ET. Note: ring of fire appearance. Typical of rheumatoid arthritis and psoriatic arthritis

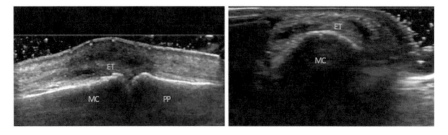

Fig. 81 **a** Longitudinal scan of the MCPJ showing (ET) extensor tendon without doppler activity and **b** Transverse scan of MCPJ showing tenosynovitis of the ET. Typical of rheumatoid arthritis and psoriatic arthritis

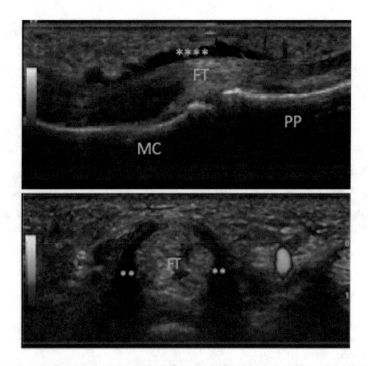

Fig. 82 a Longitudinal scan of the volar MCPJ showing tenosynovitis **** of the (FT) flexor tendon and **b** Transverse scan of MCPJ (FT) flexor tendon tenosynovitis. ** showing tenosynovitis around the tendon. Typical of rheumatoid arthritis and psoriatic arthritis

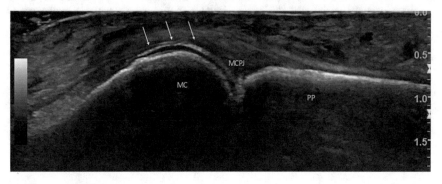

Fig. 83 Longitudinal scan of MCPJ showing double contour sign (white arrows). Typical of gout

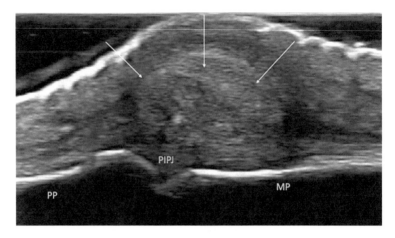

Fig. 84 Longitudinal scan of the PIPJs. Arrows point to large gouty tophi characteristic of gout

References

1. Hansen JT. Upper limb. Netter's clinical anatomy, Chapter 7, pp. 367–435. Elsevier; 2018.
2. Paulsen F. Upper extremity. In: Sobotta Atlas of Human Anatomy, Vol.1, 3, 127–242. Urban and Fischer; 2013.
3. Drake RL, Waze Vogla A, Mitchell AVM. Gray's basic anatomy, 2nd ed. Elsevier; 2017.
4. Bianchi S, Martinoli C. Ultrasound of the musculo-skeletal system. Springer; 2007.
5. Filippucci E, Iagnocco A, Meenagh G, et al. Ultrasound imaging for the rheumatologist II. Ultrasonography of the hand and wrist. Clin Exp Rheumatol. 2006;24:118–122.
6. Wakefield RJ, Balint PV, Szkudlarek M et al. OMERACT 7 Special Interest Group. Musculoskeletal ultrasound including definitions for ultrasonographic pathology. J Rheumatol. 2005;32(12):2485–7.
7. Moller I, Janta I, Backhaus M, et al. The 2017 EULAR standardized procedures for ultrasound imaging in rheumatology. Ann Rheum Dis. 2017;76(12):1974–9.

The Elbow

Iustina Janță

Anterior Elbow

For the evaluation of the anterior elbow (Illustration 1), the patient is seating facing the examiner, the elbow is extended and resting on the examination table, with the forearm supinated (Fig. 1). In some cases the elbow can be supported by a pillow.

The principal structures that can be evaluated on the anterior elbow are the radial, the coronoid and the annular recesses, the distal biceps brachii tendon and the joint cartilage.

For the evaluation of the anterior elbow, we need a linear probe with a frequency between 10 and 15 MHz.

The evaluation of the anterior elbow starts with the longitudinal view of the radial recess. The starting point is with the probe in longitudinal, just proximal to the capitellum (Fig. 2). Then the probe is swiped from medial to lateral and from proximal to distal to evaluate the radial and the annular recesses. To evaluate the coronoid recess, the probe is swiped from medial to lateral (Figs. 3 and 4). Then the probe is moved to transverse view and swiped from proximal to distal. In this scan, the radial and the coronoid recesses, the annular recess and the joint cartilage are evaluated (Figs. 5 and 6) [4].

For the evaluation of the distal biceps brachii tendon (Illustration 2), there are three approaches suggested, i.e. from anterior aspect, from medial aspect and from posterior aspect. We will discuss each approach on the corresponding aspect of the elbow. From the anterior aspect, the patient's position is the same as for the evaluation of the three anterior recesses. The probe is initially placed in longitudinal, slightly oblique, over the brachialis muscle and the radial tubercle. Slightly more pressure should be put on the distal edge of the probe (Figs. 7 and 8) [4].

I. Janță (✉)
University Hospital Valladolid, Valladolid, Spain
e-mail: iustinajanta@yahoo.com

© The Author(s), under exclusive license to Springer Nature Switzerland AG 2021   63
Q. Akram and S. Basu (eds.), *Ultrasound in Rheumatology*,
https://doi.org/10.1007/978-3-030-68659-8_3

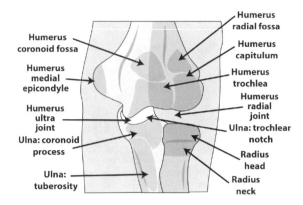

Humerus
radial fossa

Humerus
coronoid fossa

Humerus
capitulum

Humerus
medial
epicondyle

Humerus
trochlea

Humerus
radial
joint

Humerus
ultra
joint

Ulna: trochlear
notch

Ulna: coronoid
process

Ulna:
tuberosity

Radius
head

Radius
neck

Illustration 1 Anterior elbow. Figure commissioned by Dr Akram and printed with permission from Unzag Designs

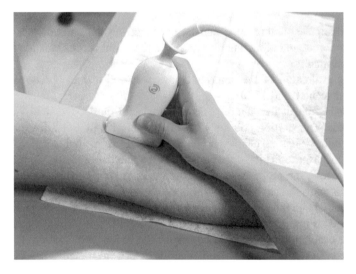

Fig. 1 Patient position and probe position (starting point) for the longitudinal evaluation of radial and annular recesses

Other structures that can be evaluated from the anterior part are the median nerve and the radial nerve. The median nerve lies medial to the brachial artery and the radial nerve lies between the brachialis medially and brachioradialis and extensor carpi radials longus laterally.

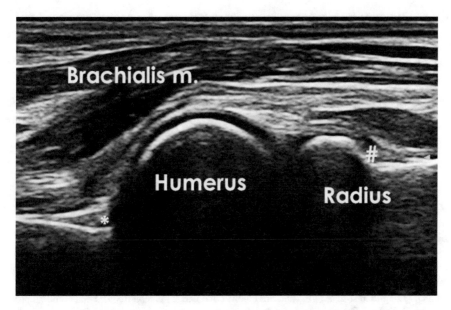

Fig. 2 Longitudinal scan of the anterior elbow. Landmarks: humeral capitellum and radial head and neck. * Radial recess; # annular recess

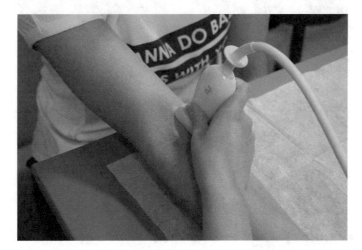

Fig. 3 Patient position and probe position (starting point) for the longitudinal evaluation of coronoid recess

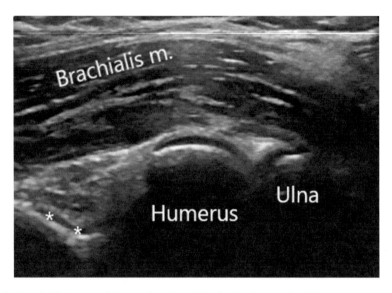

Fig. 4 Longitudinal scan of the anterior elbow. Landmarks: humeral trochlea and coronoid process of the ulna. * Coronoid recess

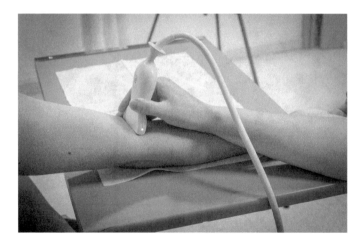

Fig. 5 Patient position and probe position (starting point) for the transverse evaluation of the anterior elbow

Medial Elbow

For the evaluation of the medial elbow, the patient is seating facing the examiner, the elbow is slightly flexed and resting on the examination table with the arm in external rotation and forearm supinated (Fig. 9) [4].

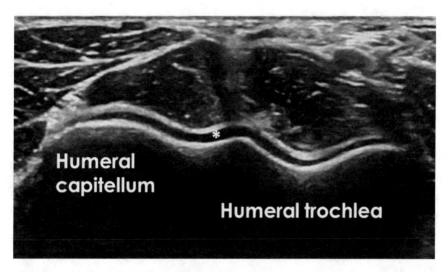

Fig. 6 Transverse scan of the anterior elbow. Landmarks: humeral capitellum and humeral trochlea. * Joint cartilage

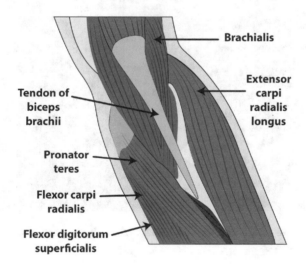

Illustration 2 Anatomical illustration of the anterior elbow including the biceps tendon. Figure commissioned by Dr Akram and printed with permission from Unzag Designs

The principal structures that can be evaluated on the medial elbow are the common flexor tendon and enthesis and the ulnar (medial) collateral ligament (Illustration 3).

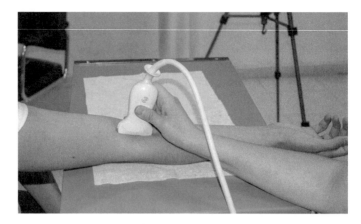

Fig. 7 Patient position and probe position (starting point) for the longitudinal evaluation of the distal biceps brachii tendon, anterior aproach

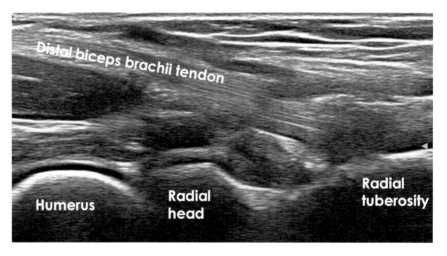

Fig. 8 Longitudinal scan of the anterior approach of the distal biceps brachii tendon. Landmarks: radial tuberosity

For the evaluation of the common flexor tendon, a high frequency, liner probe is needed (e.g. frequency more than 15 MHz).

The evaluation of the medial elbow starts with the longitudinal view of the common flexor tendon. The starting point is with the probe in longitudinal with the proximal part over the medial epicondyle and the distal part over the ulna (Fig. 10) [4]. Then the probe is swiped from medial to lateral to evaluate the entire aspect of the tendon. For the evaluation of the common flexor enthesis the probe should be moved distally, avoiding the anisotropy.

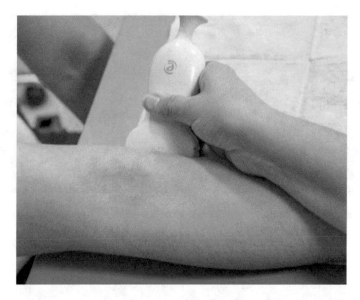

Fig. 9 Patient position and probe position (starting point) for the longitudinal evaluation of the medial elbow

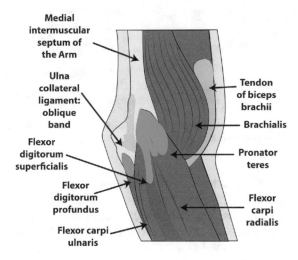

Illustration 3 Anatomical illustration of the medial elbow: common flexors

For the evaluation of biceps tendon from the medial aspect, the patient's position remains the same as for the anterior evaluation, adding that the examiner holds the patient's wrist with her/his free hand in order to perform a slightly forced external rotation (Fig. 11). The starting point is with the probe longitudinally

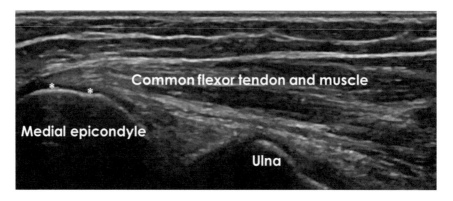

Fig. 10 Longitudinal scan of the common flexor tendon. Landmarks: medial epicondyle, proximal ulna. * Common flexor enthesis

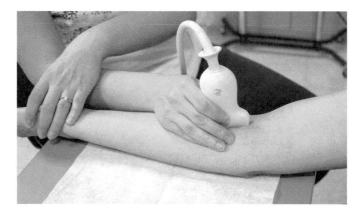

Fig. 11 Patient position and probe position (starting point) for the longitudinal evaluation of the distal biceps brachii tendon, medial aproach

and parallel to the distal humerus, with the proximal aspect of the probe over the medial epicondyle. From this point, the probe is moved distally over the pronator teres muscle, until the radial head and then the radial tuberosity is found.

The ulnar (medial) collateral ligament is a triangular ligament arising from the medial epicondyle of the humerus and inserting on to the coronoid process and olecranon of the ulna. It is formed from three bands, anterior, posterior and oblique, the anterior band being the strongest one (Fig. 12) [4].

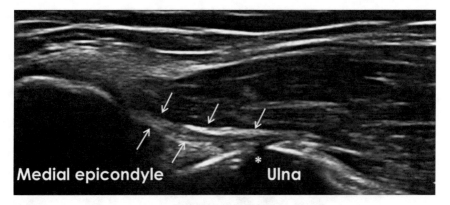

Fig. 12 Longitudinal scan of the ulnar (medial) collateral ligament (anterior band) between arrows. Landmark: medial epicondyle, ulna. * Joint space

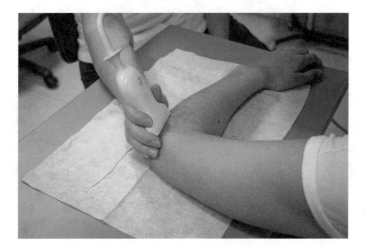

Fig. 13 Patient position and probe position (starting point) for the longitudinal evaluation of the lateral elbow

Lateral Elbow

For the evaluation of the lateral elbow, the patient is seating facing the examiner, the elbow is slightly flexed and resting on the examination table with shoulder in internal rotation (Fig. 13) [4].

The principal structures that can be evaluated on the lateral elbow are the common extensor tendon and enthesis and the radial (lateral) collateral ligament (Illustration 4).

LATERAL VIEW OF COMMON
EXTENSOR TENDON

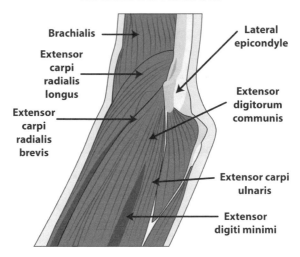

Brachialis

Extensor
carpi
radialis
longus

Extensor
carpi
radialis
brevis

Lateral
epicondyle

Extensor
digitorum
communis

Extensor carpi
ulnaris

Extensor
digiti minimi

Illustration 4   Anatomical illustration of the lateral elbow: common extensors. Figure commissioned by Dr Akram and printed with permission from Unzag Designs

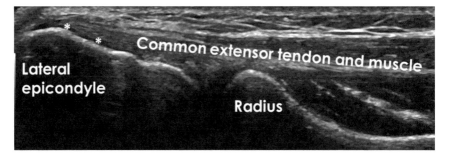

Fig. 14 Longitudinal scan of the common extensor tendon. Landmarks: lateral epicondyle, radius. * Common extensor enthesis

Due to the superficial localization of the extensor tendons, a high frequency, liner probe is needed (e.g. frequency more than 15 MHz).

The evaluation of the lateral elbow starts with the longitudinal view of the common extensor tendon.

The starting point is with the probe in longitudinal with the proximal part over the lateral epicondyle and the distal part over the radius. Then the probe is swiped from medial to lateral to evaluate the entire aspect of the tendon. For the evaluation of the common extensor enthesis, the probe should be moved distally, avoiding the anisotropy (Fig. 14) [4].

The radial (lateral) collateral ligament is weaker than the ulnar collateral ligament. It arises from the lateral epicondyle of the humerus and inserts on to the

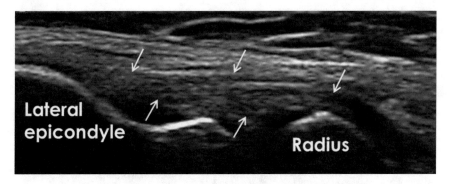

Fig. 15 Longitudinal scan of the radial (lateral) collateral ligament between arrows. Landmarks: lateral epicondyle, radial head

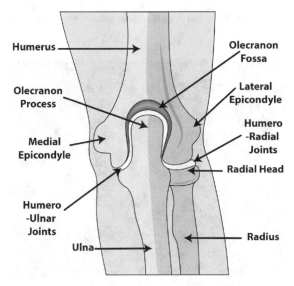

Illustration 5 Anatomical illustration of the posterior elbow. Figure commissioned by Dr Akram and printed with permission from Unzag Designs

radial notch of ulna and annular ligament. For the evaluation of the radial collateral ligament, the probe is placed in the same position as for the evaluation of the extensor tendons and swiped slightly posterior (Fig. 15) [4].

Posterior Elbow

For the evaluation of the posterior elbow, the patient is seating facing the examiner, elbow flexed and arm internally rotated, with forearm and palm resting on the examination table (Fig. 16). An alternative position is with the patient supine and the forearm and palm resting on the patient's chest [4].

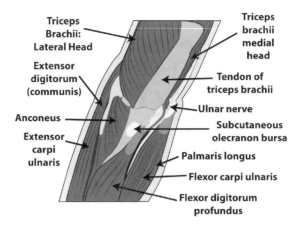

Illustration 6 Anatomical illustration of the posterior elbow including the triceps tendon. Figure commissioned by Dr Akram and printed with permission from Unzag Designs

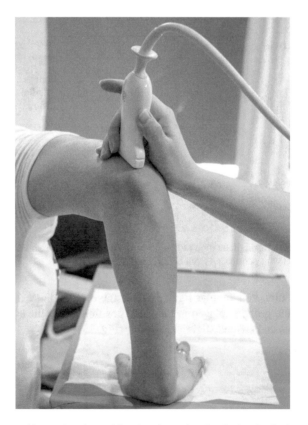

Fig. 16 Patient position and probe position (starting point) for the longitudinal evaluation of the posterior elbow

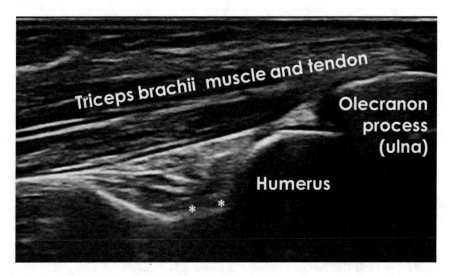

Fig. 17 Longitudinal scan of the posterior recess of the elbow. Landmark: olecranon. * Posterior recess

The principal structures that can be evaluated on the posterior elbow are the posterior joint recess and the triceps brachii tendon and enthesis (Illustrations 5 and 6).

For the evaluation of the triceps enthesis, a high frequency, liner probe is needed (e.g. frequency more than 15 MHz). On the contrary, for the evaluation of the posterior joint recess, a low frequency is needed (e.g. 10 MHz).

The starting point is with the probe placed longitudinal over the midline of the posterior proximal elbow. Then the probe is swiped from medial to lateral and from proximal to distal in order to evaluate the structures on their entire length (Figs. 17 and 18). Then the probe is moved to transverse view and swiped from proximal to distal to evaluate the posterior recess and the triceps tendon (Figs. 19 and 20) [4].

For the posterior approach for the evaluation of the biceps tendon, the patient's position is with the elbow flexed at 90 degrees, resting on the examination table, the forearm is elevated and the hand in neutral position. The starting point is with the probe transverse over the olecranon (Figs. 21 and 22). From this point, the probe is moved distally along the posterior aspect of the forearm. Dynamic manoeuvres of prono-supination are needed in order to identify the distal part of the biceps tendon and its insertion [4].

The annular ligament is the principal stabilizer of the joint and it surrounds the radial head and radial notch of the ulnar. For the evaluation of the annular ligament, the patient's elbow is flexed and resting on the examination table, hand is pronated and palmar flexed (cobra position). The probe is placed transverse to the

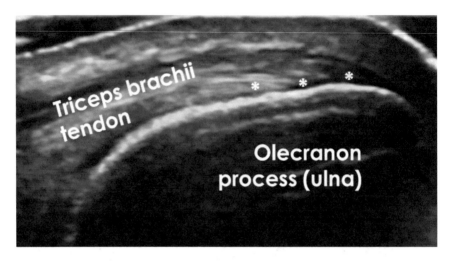

Fig. 18   Longitudinal scan of the triceps brachii tendon and enthesis (*)

radial shaft over the radial head. In this position a longitudinal view of the ligament is obtained (Fig. 23).

Other structures that can be evaluated on the posterior aspect of the elbow are
the ulnar nerve and the Osborne's ligament. For the evaluation of the ulnar nerve
in transverse view the probe is placed transverse between the olecranon and the
medial epicondyle (Figs. 24 and 25). The ulnar nerve passes in a grove, behind
the medial epicondyle. The grove is covered by the Osborne ligament, forming the
cubital tunnel. For the evaluation of the ulnar nerve subluxation dynamic maneu-
vers of flexion-extension of the elbow are useful.

Pathology

Ultrasound is useful in detecting several elbow pathologies. The evaluation of the
four recesses (i.e. the radial, the coronoid, the annular and the posterior recesses)
can detect effusion, synovitis or intraarticular bodies. The evaluation of tendons
and ligaments may detect tendinosis, enthesopathy or tears. Nerves can also be
assessed by ultrasound for entrapment, subluxation or tumours. An added value of
the ultrasound is the possibility of dynamic manoeuvres with a better characterisa-
tion of the pathology [5, 6]. If pathological finding, ultrasound has the advantage
of guiding invasive procedures.

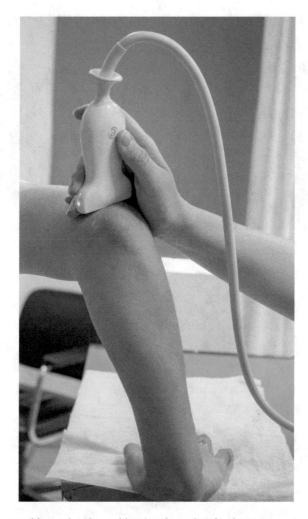

Fig. 19 Patient position and probe position (starting point) for the transverse evaluation of the posterior elbow

Synovitis is seen as an abnormal hypoechoic intra-articular tissue that is not displaceable and poorly compressible and which can exhibit Doppler sign (Fig. 26, 27, 28, 29, 30, and 31) [7]. It can be observed in several pathological settings, like rheumatoid arthritis, spondilarthropathies, crystal arthropathies and trauma. The posterior recess is the most sensitive area for the assessment of synovitis and/or joint effusion. Pathologies associated with elbow synovitis are

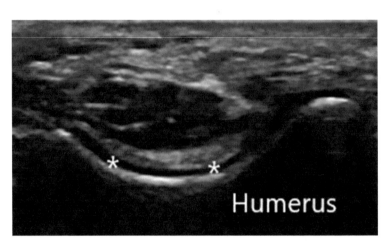

Fig. 20 Transverse scan of the posterior elbow. * Olecranon recess

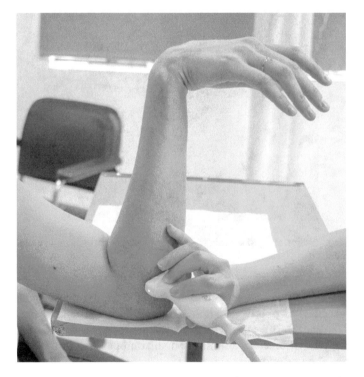

Fig. 21 Patient position and probe position (starting point) for the longitudinal evaluation of the distal biceps brachii tendon, posterior aproach

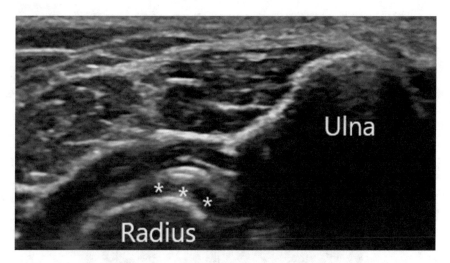

Fig. 22 Longitudinal scan of the posterior approach of the distal biceps brachii tendon. Landmark: radial and ulnar bones

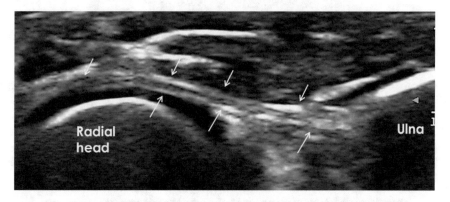

Fig. 23 Longitudinal scan of the annular ligament between arrows. Landmark: radial head

inflammatory arthritis, osteoarthrosis, crystal arthopathies, infections, pigmented villonodular synovitis or osteochrondomatosis.

Epicondylitis is mostly characterised on ultrasound by the presence of tendinopathy and/or enthesopathy. It could be caused by mechanical overuse or trauma, or by persistent inflammation. Tendinopathy appears on ultrasound as focal or generalized hypoechogenicity with or without Doppler sign. In mechanical pathologies, the presence of Doppler sign is due to regenerative tendon response

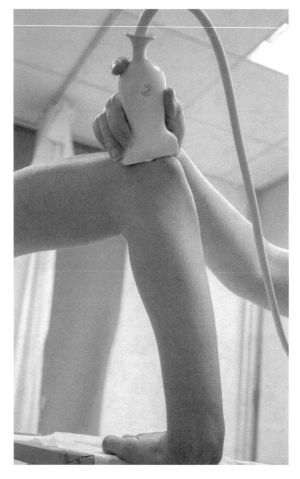

Fig. 24 Patient position and probe position (starting point) for the transverse evaluation of the ulnar nerve

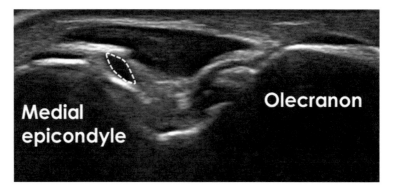

Fig. 25 Transverse scan of the ulnar nerve (dash line). Landmark: medial epicondyle

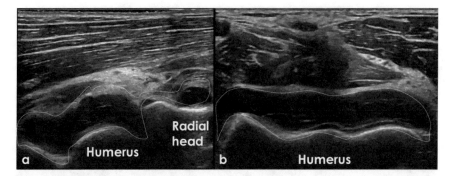

Fig. 26 Longitudinal and transverse view of radial and annular recesses showing synovitis (dash line)

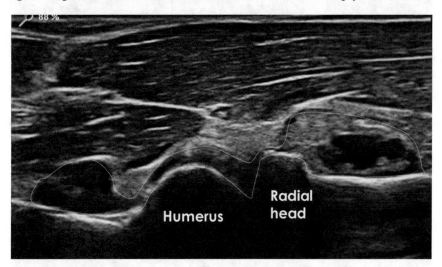

Fig. 27 Longitudinal view of radial and annular recesses showing synovitis (dash line)

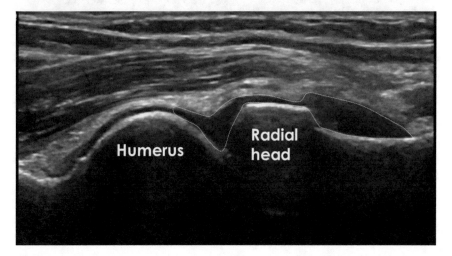

Fig. 28 Longitudinal view of annular recess showing synovitis (dash line)

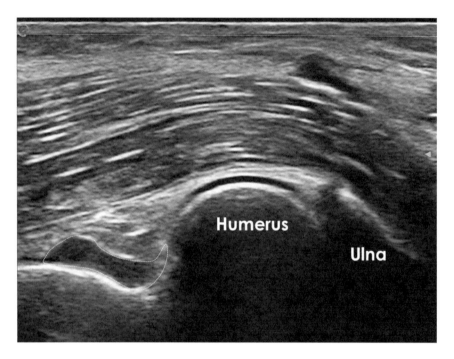

Fig. 29 Longitudinal view of coronoid recess showing synovitis (dash line)

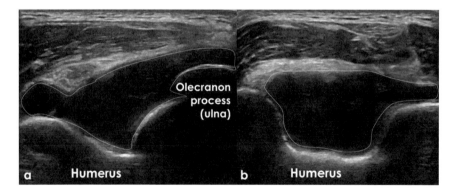

Fig. 30 (**a, b**) Longitudinal and transverse view of the posterior recess showing synovitis (dash line)

(Fig. 32a,b). Mechanical tendinopathy is more frequent at the extensor tendons levels, compared to medial flexor tendons.

Entesopathy is defined as an abnormal hyperechoic (loss of normal fibrillary architecture) and/or thickened tendon at its bony attachment. Others findings, like enthesophytes, erosions or calcifications can be observed. Ultrasound enthesitis

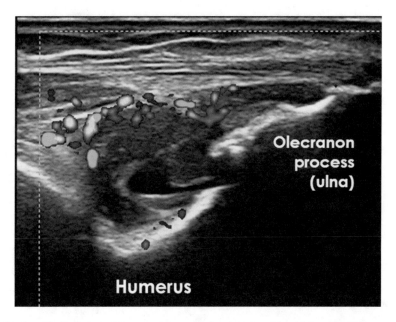

Fig. 31 Longitudinal view of the posterior recess showing synovitis with Doppler sign

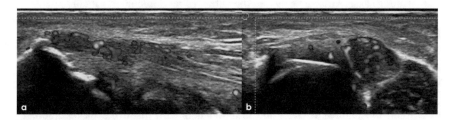

Fig. 32 (a,b). Longitudinal and transverse view of the extensor tendons showing tendinopathy with Doppler sign

is defined by the Outcome Measures in Rheumatology (OMERACT) group as "hypoechoic and/or thickened insertion of the tendon close to the bone (within 2 mm from the bony cortex), which exhibits Doppler signal if active and that may show erosions, enthesophytes/calcifications as a sign of structural damage" (Fig. 33) [8]. According to this definition, the presence of inflammatory signs (i.e. Doppler sign and/or hypoechoic and/or thickened tendon insertion) is mandatory to define enthesitis in spondilarthropathies (i.e. spondyloarthtitis and psoriatic arthritis).

Clinically, it may be difficult to differentiate between tendinopathy/entesopathy and enthesitis. Thus, ultrasound may be used to identify the presence of enthesitis,

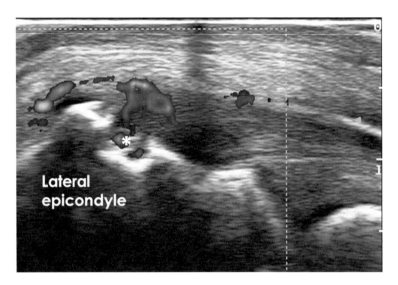

Fig. 33 Longitudinal view of the extensor tendons showing enthesitis with Doppler sign and erosion (*)

features more specific for espondilarthropathy. On the other hand, ultrasound it is also useful to assess the severity and the extent of tendon/enthesis involvement.

At the elbow level, the most frequently involved bursae are the olecranon and bicipital bursae. The normal bursae are not visible, but in some pathological situations, like crystal arthopathies, infections, repetitive trauma or inflammatory arthritis, they are distended and can be easily observed (Fig. 34). For a better visualization of this bursitis, it is important not to put too much pressure on the probe, especially for the olecranon bursitis. The bicipital bursitis is frequently due to chronic mechanical friction and is associated with distal biceps tendinopathy (Figs. 35 and 36a,b).

Although it is not the most symptomatic joint in crystal arthropaties, crystal deposits of uric acid and calcium pyrophosphate can be observed at the elbow joint. For uric acid deposits, the most frequent finding is the presence of tophi at the olecranon burse or within the triceps tendon (Fig. 37); the double contour sign may be also observed. Calcium pyrophosphate deposits may be observed as hyperechoic images within the joint cartilage (Fig. 38).

Tendon and ligament tears may be observed as an anechoic or hypoechoic discontinuity of the fibrillary pattern with or without retraction and, in recent cases, with surrounding hypoechoic fluid. The most frequent tendon tears at the elbow

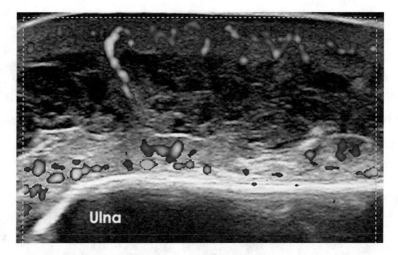

Fig. 34 Longitudinal view over the proximal ulna showing olecranon bursitis

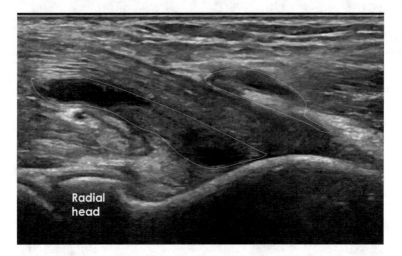

Fig. 35 Longitudinal view of the distal brachii tendon showing bicipital bursitis (dash line)

level are those involving the distal biceps brachii tendon, although, these tears are much less common than the proximal biceps brachii tears. Regarding the elbow ligaments, the ulnar collateral ligament is most frequently involved.

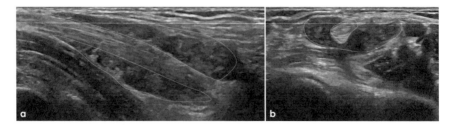

Fig. 36 (**a**, **b**) Longitudinal and transverse view of the distal brachii tendon showing bicipital bursitis

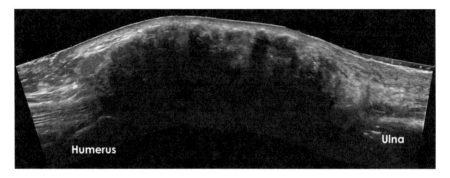

Fig. 37 Extended longitudinal view of the posterior elbow showing a hyperechoic image with acoustic shadow (tophi)

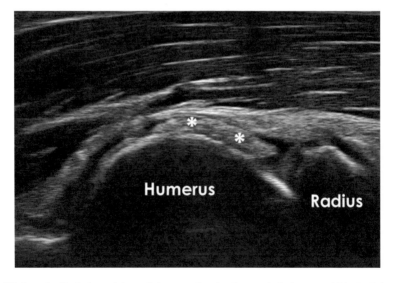

Fig. 38 Longitudinal view of the radial recess showing hyperechoic images within the joint cartilage (*)

References

1. Elbow and forearm. Susan Standring MBE. In: Gray's anatomy, Chapter 49. p. 837–61.e3.
2. Hansen JT. Upper limb. In: Netter's clinical anatomy, Chapter 7. p. 367–435.
3. Paulsen F. Upper extremity. In: Sobotta atlas of human anatomy, vol. 1, no. 3. p. 127–242.
4. Moller I, Janta I, Backhaus M, et al. The 2017 EULAR standardized procedures for ultrasound imaging in rheumatology. Ann Rheum Dis. 2017;76(12):1974–9.
5. Draghi F, et al. Ultrasound of the elbow: examination techniques and US appearance of the normal and pathologic joint. J Ultrasound. 2007;10:76–84.
6. Konin GP, Nazarian LN, Walz DM. US of the elbow: indications, technique, normal anatomy, and pathologic conditions. Radiographics. 2013;33(4):E125–47.
7. Wakefield RJ, Balint PV, Szkudlarek M et al. OMERACT 7 Special Interest Group. Musculoskeletal ultrasound including definitions for ultrasonographic pathology. J Rheumatol. 2005;32(12):2485–87.
8. Terslev L, Naredo E, Iagnocco A, et al. Defining enthesitis in spondyloarthritis by ultrasound: results of a Delphi process and of a reliability reading exercise, Outcome Measures in Rheumatology Ultrasound Task Force. Arthritis Care Res. 2004;66:741–8.

The Shoulder

Subhasis Basu

Basic Anatomy

The shoulder joint consists of the larger glenohumeral joint and smaller acromio-humeral joint which is located more superiorly. Ultrasound is not well established at evaluating the intra-articular structures however good visualisation to the posterior glenohumeral joint is appreciable which is useful to assess for any joint effusions as well as partial view of the humeral chondral surfaces and the posterior labrum. The acromiohumeral joint is well seen in both longitudinal and transverse planes and can prove useful to assess for degenerative features or joint effusions. Dynamic assessment to look for joint instability can also be performed particularly if you can compare with the contralateral and un-injured joint.

There are 4 main tendons that make up the rotator cuff muscles which including the subscapularis (anterior), supraspinatus (anterosuperior), infraspinatus (posterosuperior) and teres minor (postero-inferior). Ultrasound can identify the attachments of the tendons onto the greater and lesser tuberosities of the humeral head.

Anteriorly, the long head of biceps tendon courses along the anterior margin of the shoulder within the inter tubercular grove. The short head of biceps tendon origin is at the coracoid process. The long head of biceps tendon origin is intra-articular at the supraglenoid tubercle which is less well appreciated on ultrasound compared to its extra-articular segment along the bicipital grove. Finally, nestled between the rotator cuff tendons and the overlying acromio-clavicular (AC joint) and deltoid muscle lies the subacromial/subdeltoid bursa which can be thickened or distended with fluid in the context of bursitis.

S. Basu (✉)
Consultant Musculoskeletal Radiologist, Wrightington Hospital, Wrightington, UK
e-mail: sbasu81@doctors.org.uk

© The Author(s), under exclusive license to Springer Nature Switzerland AG 2021
Q. Akram and S. Basu (eds.), *Ultrasound in Rheumatology*,
https://doi.org/10.1007/978-3-030-68659-8_4

Basic Patient Positioning and Imaging Protocol

When examining the shoulder, there is no right or wrong way of positioning the patient in reality. What is most important is to ensure the patient can be as comfortable as possible during the examination with relative freedom to move the shoulder and arm as you will see below. Furthermore, it is important to ensure that as the operator performing the ultrasound study, that you are also comfortable with accessibility to the patient and performing various manoeuvres whilst scanning the patient's shoulder.

By convention, the patient is usually sat on a chair/stool with the ultrasound operator stood behind the patient with the scanner in front of you, or the examiner is sat opposite the patient rather than behind.

In order to ensure a comprehensive ultrasound study of the shoulder has been performed and in order to minimise errors and incomplete coverage, it is suggested that a scanning protocol is adhered to each time to ensure standardisation.

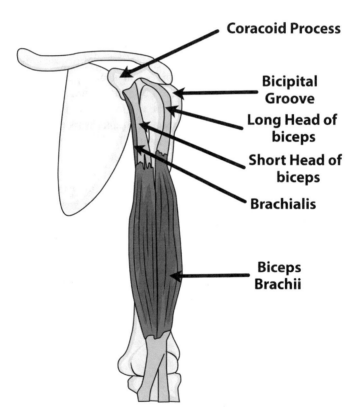

Illustration 1 Schematic highlighting the portion of the short and long head of the biceps tendon and biceps brachii muscle along the anterior upper arm. Figure commissioned by Dr Akram and printed with permission from Unzag Designs

In order to scan the shoulder structures, a linear array probe with a high frequency is suggested e.g. 12–15 MHz transducer. This allows for better resolution with a balance between depth and penetration. You must also be aware that patients with differing body habitus could mean that to optimise imaging, you may need to change your transducer to a lower frequency linear array transducer to ensure you get adequate depth and penetration without losing out too much on image resolution. Ensure that adequate depth and focus is used with one hand controlling and optimising the ultrasound settings, whilst the other is used to scan the relevant regions around the shoulder.

The protocol outlined below involves starting to scan the shoulder anteriorly, followed by anterosuperiorly, posterosuperiorly and finally posteroinferiorly.

Anteriorly, the structures to be scanned include the long head of biceps (Illustration 1) and subscapularis tendons (Illustration 2). Then as we move anterosuperiorly, we include the rotator interval followed by the supraspinatus tendon and subacromial bursa (Illustration 3). Then we move to the AC joint (Illustration 4) followed by the infraspinatus and teres minor tendons posteriorly and postero-inferiorly. Finally, the examination is completed by evaluating the posterior glenohumeral joint (Illustration 5).

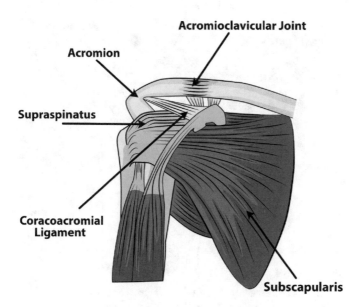

Illustration 2 Schematic highlighting the anterior subscapularis muscle and its tendon fibres inserting into the lesser tuberosity footplate and overlying the long head of biceps tendon. Figure commissioned by Dr Akram and printed with permission from Unzag Designs

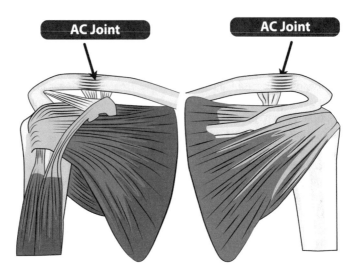

Illustration 3 Schematic highlighting the superior position of the AC joint in both anterior (left) and posterior (right) views. Figure commissioned by Dr Akram and printed with permission from Unzag Designs

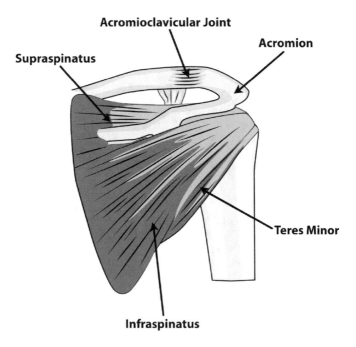

Illustration 4 Schematic highlighting the posterior rotator cuff muscles and tendons. Figure commissioned by Dr Akram and printed with permission from Unzag Designs

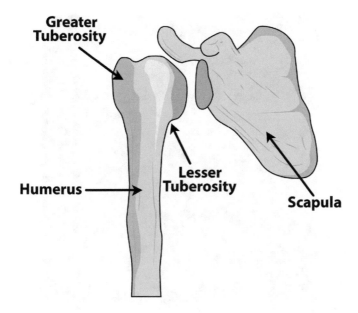

Illustration 5 Schematic highlighting the posterior aspect of the glenohumeral joint. Figure commissioned by Dr Akram and printed with permission from Unzag Designs

Anterior Structures

The examination of the shoulder starts with a scan of the long head of biceps tendon.

The patient's hand should be resting on the ipsilateral thigh with the elbow flexed at 90 degrees. The transducer is placed in a transverse plane in the biciptal groove (Figs. 1 and 2). The transducer should slide cranio-caudally to examine the entire length of the long head biceps tendon. Caudally, you should scan the tendon to its musculotendinous junction.

The transducer is then rotated 180 degrees and a longitudinal view of the biceps tendon is seen (Figs. 3 and 4).

The patient is then asked to externally rotate the arm whilst keeping the elbow flexed at 90 degrees and the transducer is initially placed in a transverse position over the lesser tuberosity of the humerus (Figs. 5 and 6). The probe is then rotated 180 degrees to view the subscapularis tendon in a longitudinal view (Figs. 7 and 8).

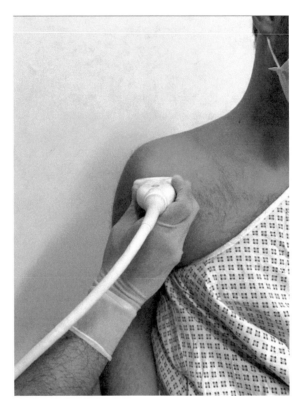

Fig. 1 Patient position and probe position (starting point) for the transverse evaluation of the the proximal bicipital groove to view the long head of biceps tendon

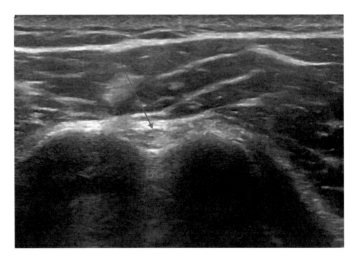

Fig. 2 Transverse view of the long head of biceps tendon within the bicipital groove. Red arrow = biceps tendon. BG = bicipital groove

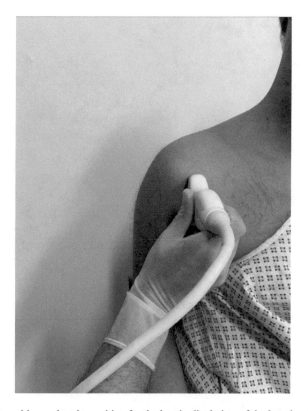

Fig. 3 Patient position and probe position for the longitudinal view of the long head of biceps tendon

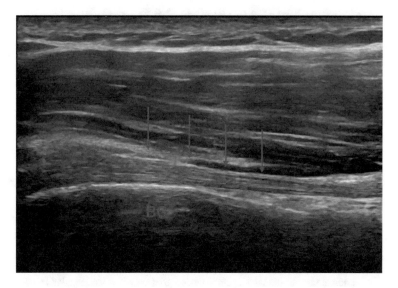

Fig. 4 Longitudinal view of the long head of biceps tendon within the bicipital groove. Red arrows = biceps tendon. BG = bicipital groove

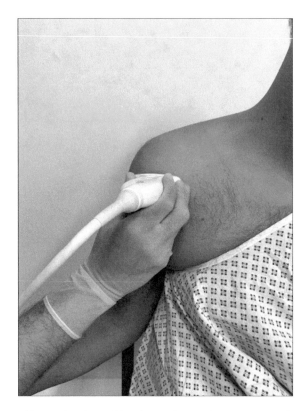

Fig. 5 Patient position and probe position for the longitudinal evaluation of the subscapularis tendon

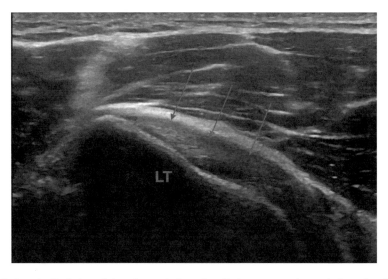

Fig. 6 Longitudinal view of the subscapularis tendon. Red arrows = subscapularis tendon. LT = lesser tuberosity

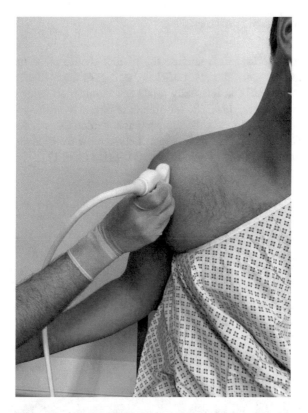

Fig. 7 Patient position and probe position for the transverse evaluation of the subscapularis tendon

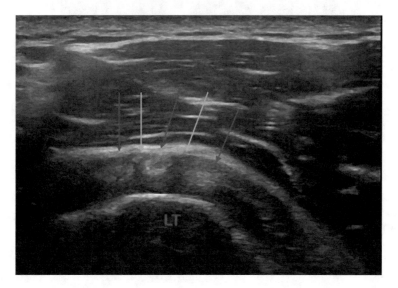

Fig. 8 Transverse view of subscapularis tendon with the characteristic normal striated hypo-echoic and hyper-echoic appearance to the myofascicular structure. Red arrows = hyperechoic tendon bundles. Green arrows = hypoechoic muscle fibres. LT = lesser tuberosity

Anterosuperior Structures

To examine the supraspinatus tendon, the patient should place their arm behind their back and also place the palm of their hand onto the ipsilateral back pocket. This helps to to abduct and internally rotate the shoulder allowing the supraspinatus tendon to come into view. The transducer is placed over the greater tuberosity in a transverse position to view the supraspinatus tendon (Figs. 9 and 10).

The probe can then be rotated in a longitudinal view over the greater tuberosity to view the supraspinatus tendon in long axis (Figs. 11 and 12).

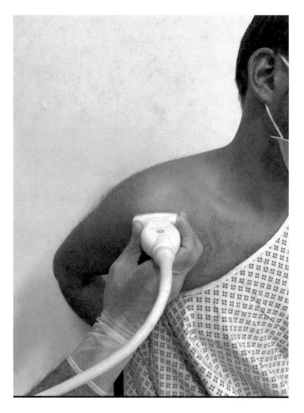

Fig. 9 Patient position and probe position for the transverse evaluation of the supraspinatus tendon

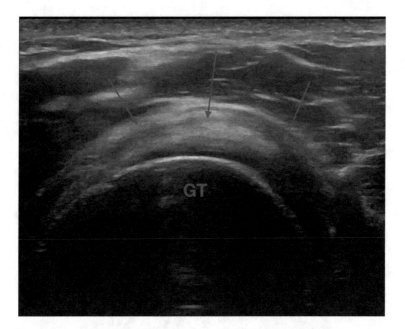

Fig. 10 Transverse view of the supraspinatus tendon. Red arrows = supraspinatus tendon. GT = greater tuberosity

Posterosuperior Structures

Scanning of the AC joint is done by placing the arm of the patient in the neutral position. The probe is placed in a longitudinal plane over the acromion process and the clavicle (Figs. 13 and 14) and then in a transverse plane (Figs. 15 and 16).

This same position can be used to dynamically examine for any clinical signs of subacromial impingement by abducting the shoulder and assessing for any 'bunching' up of the subacromial bursa with the transducer positioned over the acromion process at its most lateral aspect.

To scan the infraspinatus tendon, teres minor tendon and posterior gleno-humeral joint space, the patient's arm is placed across the front of their chest whilst the transducer is placed over the posterior shoulder and posterior facet of the greater tuberosity. This is also the position to access the glenohumeral joint posteriorly for either aspirations or injections.

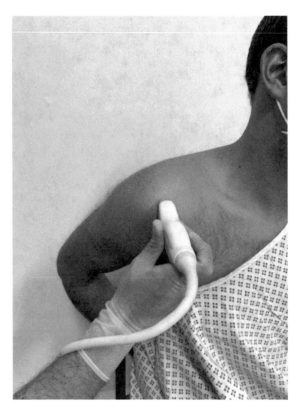

Fig. 11 Patient position and probe position for the longitudinal evaluation of the supraspinatus tendon

Figure 17 shows the longitudinal position of the transducer over the posterior facet of the greater tuberosity to view the infraspinatus and teres minor tendon insertions. The arm is forward flexed and brought across the chest wall. Figure 18 shows the longitudinal view of the infraspinatus tendon at its greater tuberosity insertion.

Figure 19 shows the longitudinal position of the transducer to view the glenohumeral joint (GHJ) posteriorly. Figure 20 shows the longitudinal view of the posterior glenohumeral joint.

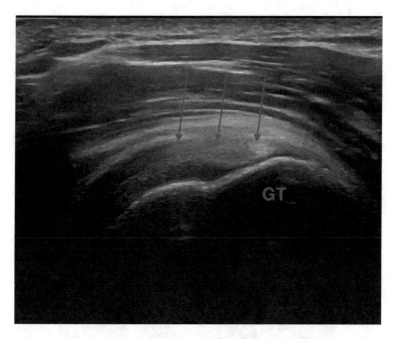

Fig. 12 Longitudinal view of the supraspinatus tendon footprint at the greater tuberosity foot-plate. Red arrows = supraspinatus tendon. GT = greater tuberosity

Pathology

Ultrasound is a great imaging modality to consider assessment for various shoulder pathology. As it is a live and dynamic examination, the ultrasound can be used as an extension in the office to complement the clinical history and examination findings, thus help narrow down your differential diagnoses.

Inflammation and excess fluid around the long head of biceps tendon can be visualised e.g. in tenosynovitis as well as dynamically examine for any biceps subluxation or dislocation (Figs. 21, 22, and 23). Fluid distension and inflammation to the overlying subacromial bursa (Figs. 23 and 24) can be assessed as well as identifying synovitis within the glenohumeral joint (Fig. 25) or the smaller acromioclavicular joint (Fig. 26).

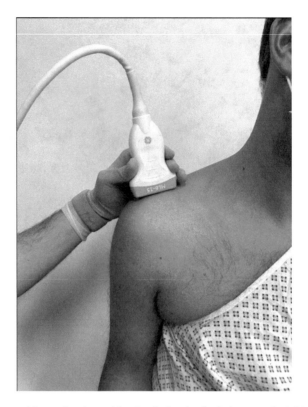

Fig. 13 Patient position and probe position for the longitudinal view over the AC joint. The arm is in neutral position

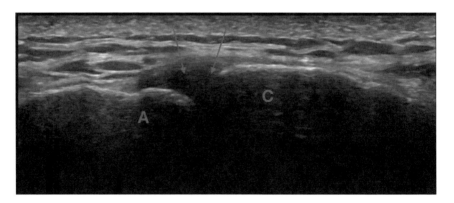

Fig. 14 Longitudinal view of the AC joint. A acromion process. C = clavicle. The red arrows = superior joint capsule

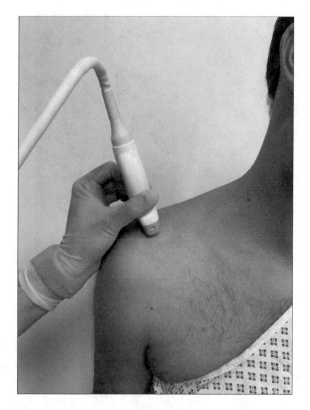

Fig. 15 Patient position and probe position for the transverse evaluation of the AC joint

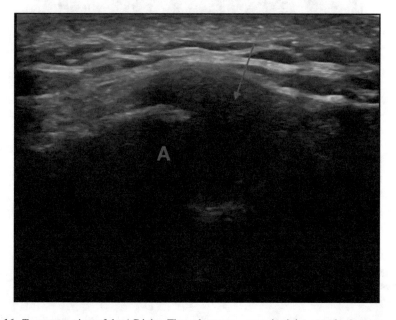

Fig. 16 Transverse view of the AC joint. The red arrows = superior joint capsule. A = acromion process seen en profile

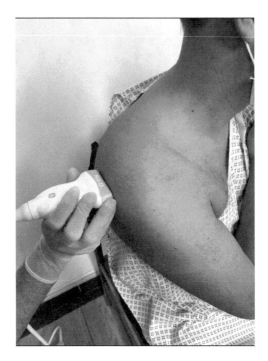

Fig. 17 Longitudinal position of the transducer over the posterior facet of the greater tuberosity to view the infraspinatus and teres minor tendon insertions

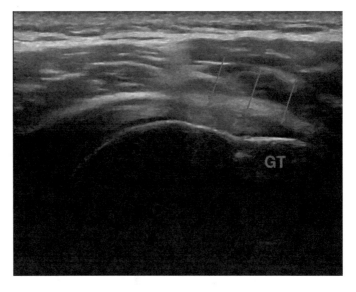

Fig. 18 Longitudinal view of the infraspinatus tendon at its greater tuberosity insertion. Red arrows = infraspinatus tendon. GT = greater tuberosity

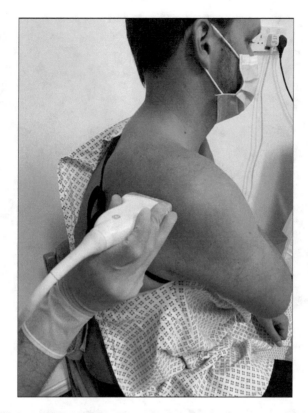

Fig. 19 Longitudinal position of the transducer to view the glenohumeral joint (GHJ) posteriorly; Also used as access to inject or aspirate from the GHJ

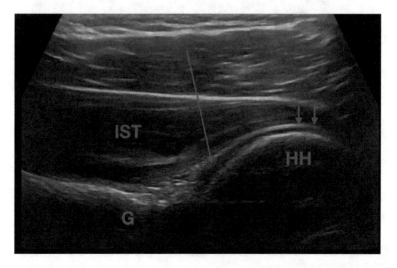

Fig. 20 Longitudinal view of the posterior glenohumeral joint. IST = infraspinatus muscle belly. G = the posterior glenoid. HH = posterior humeral head, Short red arrows = hypoechoic humeral head chondral surface. Long red arrow = hypoechoic GHJ space

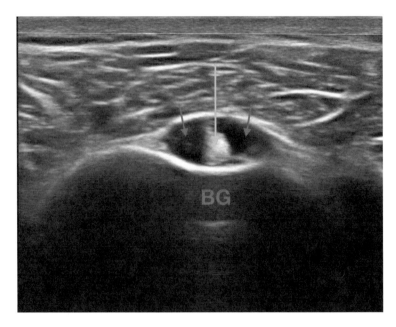

Fig. 21 Biceps tenosynovitis in transverse view. Green arrow = biceps tendon. BG = bicipital groove. Red arrow = tenosynovitis with hypoechoic fluid surrounding the biceps tendon

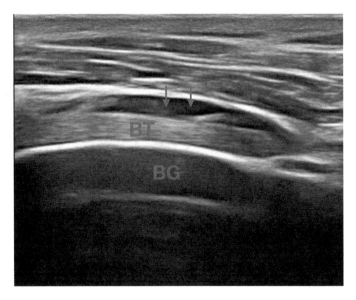

Fig. 22 Biceps tenosynovitis in longitudinal view. BT = biceps tendon. BG = bicipital groove. Red arrows = tenosynovitis

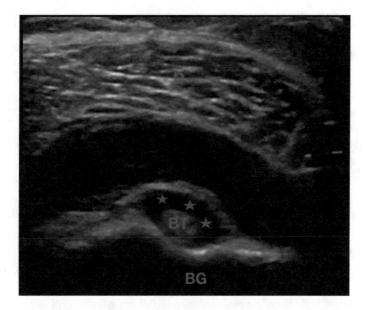

Fig. 23 Large SASD bursitis in transverse view (white arrow). BT = biceps tendon. *** is teno-synovitis around the biceps tendon (BT). BG = bicipital groove. D = deltoid muscle

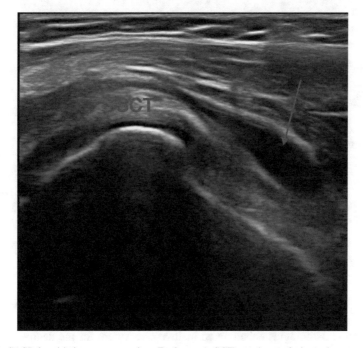

Fig. 24 SASD bursitis in transverse view (Red arrow). SCT = subscapularis tendon

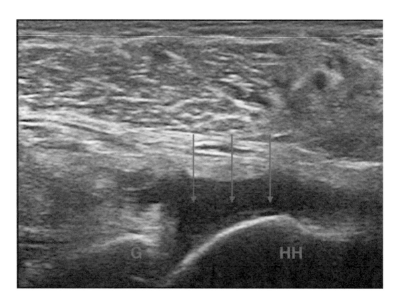

Fig. 25 Longitudinal view of the glenohumeral joint showing synovitis (Red arrows). D = deltoid muscle. G = posterior glenoid. HH = humeral head

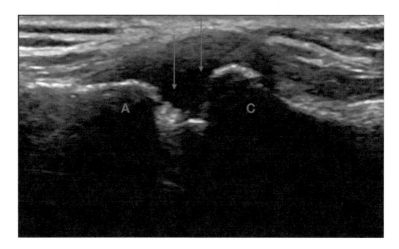

Fig. 26 Longitudinal view of the acromio-clavicular joint. Red arrow = osteophytes and adjacent synovial hypertrophy. A = acromion. C = clavicle

Calcific tendinitis is not an uncommon pathology and calcific foci within the rotator cuff tendons are easily visible (Fig. 27).

Common pathologies encountered include assessment for the degree of rotator cuff tendinopathy (Figs. 28 and 29) as well as for any superimposed partial-thickness or full-thickness cuff tears (Figs. 30, 31, and 32).

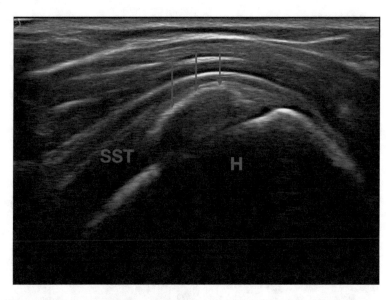

Fig. 27 Longitudinal view of (SST) supraspinatus tendon. Calcific tendinitis (Red arrows). H = humerus

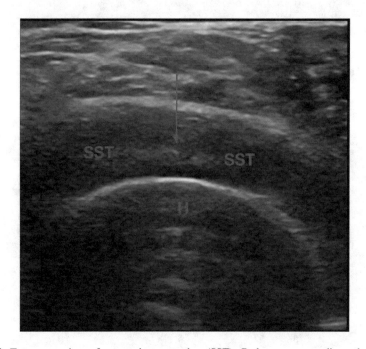

Fig. 28 Transverse view of supraspinatus tendon (SST). Red arrow = tendinopathy. H = humeral head

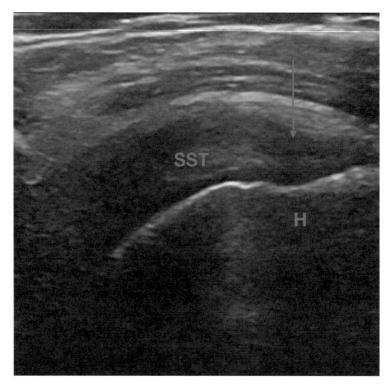

Fig. 29 Longitudinal view of supraspinatus tendon (SST). Red arrow = tendinopathy. H = humeral head

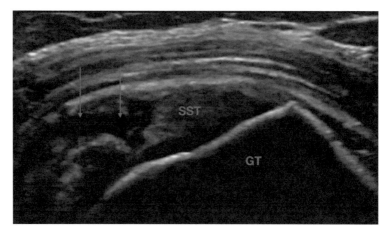

Fig. 30 Longitudinal view of (SST) supraspinatus tendon. Full thickness tear of the tendon (Red arrows). GT = greater tuberosity

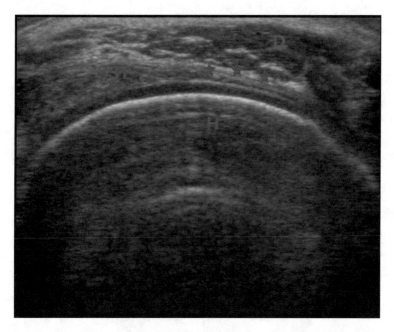

Fig. 31 Transverse view of supraspinatus tendon (SST). *** indicating complete tear of the tendon. D = deltoid muscle sagging upon the humeral head. H = humeral head

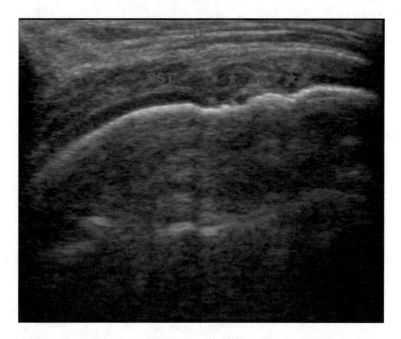

Fig. 32 Longitudinal view of supraspinatus tendon (SST). *** indicating complete tear of the tendon. D = deltoid muscle

Acknowledgements Dr. Jay Panchal—Musculoskeletal Radiology Fellow and Mr. Dean Eckersley—Superintendent Radiographer

References

1. Moller I, Janta I, Backhaus M, et al. The 2017 EULAR standardized procedures for ultrasound imaging in rheumatology. Ann Rheum Dis. 2017;76(12):1974–9.
2. Beggs I. Shoulder ultrasound. Semin Ultrasound CT MR. 2011;32(2):101–13.
3. Bianchi S, Martinoli C. Ultrasound of the musculo-skeletal system. Springer; 2007.

The Hip

Subhasis Basu

Basic Anatomy

The hip joint consists of the femoral head articulating with the acetabulum. Ultrasound is not as well established at evaluating the deeper, intra-articular structures however, good visualisation to the anterior hip joint capsule is appreciable which is useful to assess for any joint effusions, synovitis, as well as partial view of the acetabular labrum anteriorly and parts of the femoral head articular cartilage, the psoas tendon and bursa if it is distended, and the surrounding soft tissue structures.

The commonly requested tendons to be assessed around the hip tend to be the lateral hip abductors comprising of the gluteal medius and minimus tendons that insert onto the various facets of the greater trochanter.

Another tendon that can be assessed in the context of groin pain includes the psoas tendon anteriorly and any fluid distension can lead to an iliopsoas bursitis. Posteriorly the common hamstring origins can be assessed as they insert into the ischial tuberosity to look for signs of enthesopathy or tendon tears.

Basic Patient Positioning and Imaging Protocol

When examining the hip, it is important to ensure the patient can be as comfortable as possible during the examination with relative freedom to move the hip and lower leg. A comfortable patient makes it easier for the operator to scan the patient. Furthermore, it is important to ensure that as the person performing the ultrasound examination, that you are also comfortable with accessibility to the patient.

S. Basu (✉)
Wrightington Hospital, Wigan, Greater Manchester, UK
e-mail: sbasu81@doctors.org.uk

© The Author(s), under exclusive license to Springer Nature Switzerland AG 2021   113
Q. Akram and S. Basu (eds.), *Ultrasound in Rheumatology*,
https://doi.org/10.1007/978-3-030-68659-8_5

By convention, the patient is usually lying supine on an examining couch to the right of the ultrasound examiner. If the anterior hip joint and surrounding structures are being scanned, then the patient is lying supine on the couch; if the lateral hip abductor tendon insertions are examined then the patient is rolled onto their side on their contralateral hip; if the posterior muscle compartments of the hip are to be examined then the patient is turned prone onto the examining couch.

There is no absolute correct or incorrect way of scanning the various structures in and around the hip. If the main aim of the ultrasound is to answer a specific clinical question by performing a targeted examination, then you may proceed to scan that structure(s). In order to ensure a comprehensive ultrasound study of the hip has been performed and minimise errors and incomplete coverage, it is suggested that a scanning protocol is devised and adhered to each time to ensure standardisation and consistency.

The protocol outlined below involves starting to scan the hip anteriorly (Figs. 1, 2, 3, 4 and Illustration 1), followed by laterally (Figs. 5, 6, 7, 8 and Illustration 2) and then posteriorly (Figs. 9, 10, 11, 12, 13, 14 and Illustration 3). The groin region can then be imaged medially (Figs. 15, 16, 17, 18). In order to scan the hip structures, a linear array probe with lower frequency is suggested e.g. a 9–14 MHz transducer. This allows for better resolution with adequate depth penetration. You must also be aware that patients with differing body habitus could mean that to optimise imaging, you may need to change your transducer to an even lower

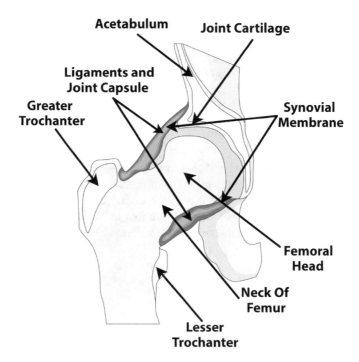

Illustration 1 Illustration highlighting the hip joint and surrounding soft tissue structures. Figure commissioned by Dr Akram and printed with permission from Unzag Designs

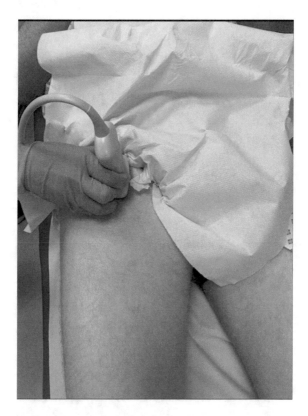

Fig. 1 Patient position and probe position (starting point) for the scanning of the anterior hip joint and capsule in a long axis view

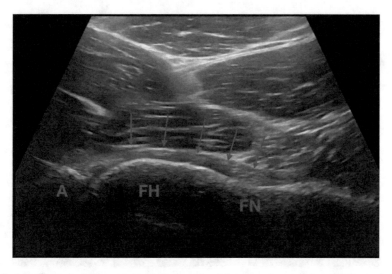

Fig. 2 Longitudinal oblique view of the anterior joint capsule overlying the femoral head and neck. FH—femoral head. FN—femoral neck. The anterior joint capsule is outlined by red arrows. A—acetabulum

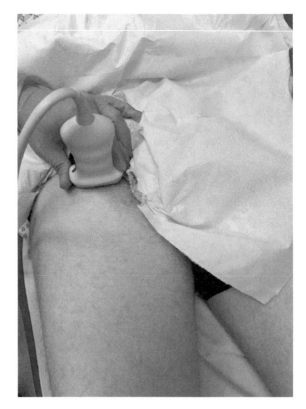

Fig. 3 Transverse transducer position over the femoral head. FH—femoral head. The joint capsule is outlined by red arrows

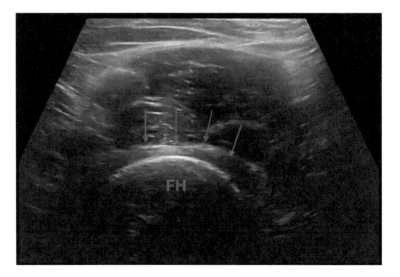

Fig. 4 Transverse view of the anterior joint capsule overlying the femoral head

frequency curvilinear transducer to ensure you get adequate depth penetration without losing out too much on image resolution. Ensure that adequate depth and focus is maintained, with one hand used to control the ultrasound machine and its settings, whilst the other is used to scan the relevant regions in and around the hip.

Anterior Structures

The examination of the hip starts with the anterior hip joint and capsule. The patient lies supine with the transducer placed obliquely over the femoral neck to examine the entire length of the joint and sweeping from side-to-side (Figs. 1 and 2). Following this, the probe is placed in a transverse position over the femoral head (Figs. 3 and 4). Illustration 1 highlights the hip joint and surrounding structures.

Lateral Structures

Illustration 2 shows the anatomy of the lateral hip joint.

The patient is lying on their side in a lateral decubitus position onto the contralateral hip. The transducer is placed in a longitudinal axis over the greater trochanter (Figs. 5 and 6).

The probe is then rotated 180 degrees to obtain a transverse view of the abductor tendons over the greater trochanter (Figs. 7 and 8).

Posterior Structures

To scan the posterior structures the patient is asked to lie prone on the couch. Illustration 3 highlights the relevant posterior hip and thigh structures.

The transducer is placed in a transverse view over the ischial tuberosity (Fig. 9) and a transverse view of the hamstring tendon is obtained (Fig. 10). The probe is then rotated (Fig. 11) and a longitudinal view of the hamstring origin is obtained (Fig. 12).

The probe can then be rotated again and swept inferiorly over the mid thigh to obtain a view of the hamstring muscles (Figs. 13 and 14).

Medial Structures

Finally, the medial structures can be examined. Ask the patient to lie supine with the hip abducted and the ipsilateral knee mildly flexed.

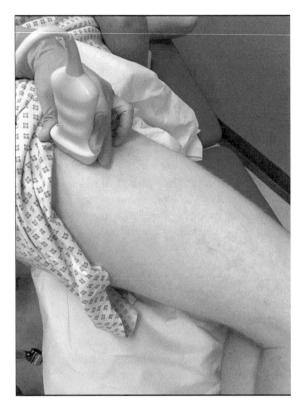

Fig. 5 Longitudinal transducer position over the greater trochanter with the patient lying in the lateral decubitus position on their contralateral side

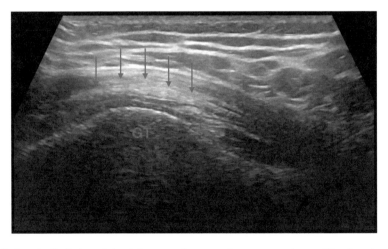

Fig. 6 Longitudinal view of the abductor tendons over the greater trochanter. The gluteal medius tendon is outlined by the red arrows. GT—greater trochanter

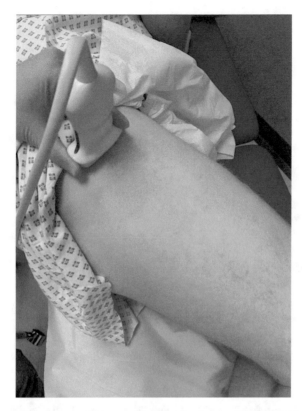

Fig. 7 Transverse transducer position over the greater trochanter with patient lying in the lateral decubitus position on their contralateral hip

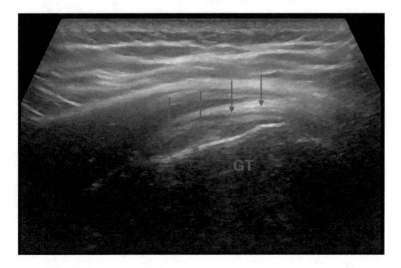

Fig. 8 Transverse view of the abductor tendons over the greater trochanter. The gluteal medius tendon is outlined by the red arrows. GT—greater trochanter

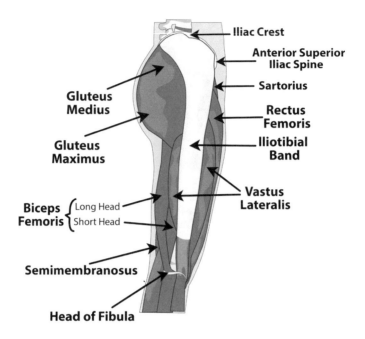

Illustration 2 Ilustration highlighting the principal anterior, posterior and lateral muscles around the hip. Figure commissioned by Dr Akram and printed with permission from Unzag Designs

Initially, the probe is placed in a longitudinal plane in an oblique position over the adductor muscles whilst the hip is abducted and knee flexed (Fig. 15) to obtain a view of the adductor muscle group converging onto the pubis.

The probe is then placed in a transverse position to obtain the short axis view (Figs. 17 and 18).

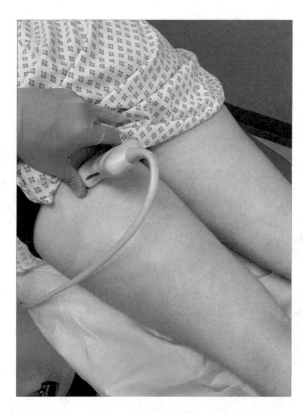

Fig. 9 Transverse transducer position over ischial tuberosity with patient lying prone on the couch

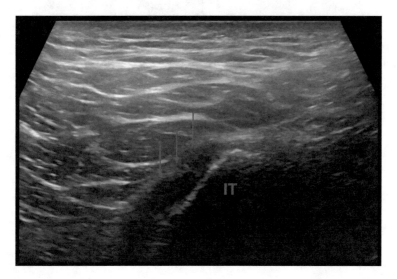

Fig. 10 Transverse view of the hamstring origin at the ischial tuberosity. IT—ischial tuberosity. The common hamstring origin tendons are outlined by red arrows

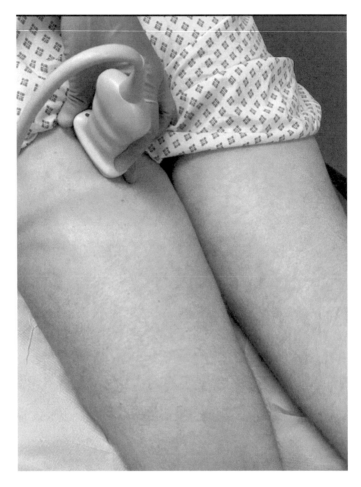

Fig. 11 Longitudinal transducer position of the hamstring origin at the ischial tuberosity with the patient lying prone

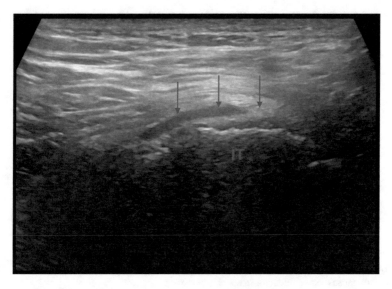

Fig. 12 Longitudinal view of the hamstring origin at the ischial tuberosity. IT—ischial tuberosity. The common hamstring origin tendons are outlined by red arrows

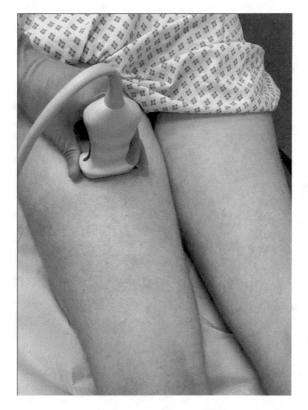

Fig. 13 Transverse transducer position over the mid posterior thigh with the patient lying prone

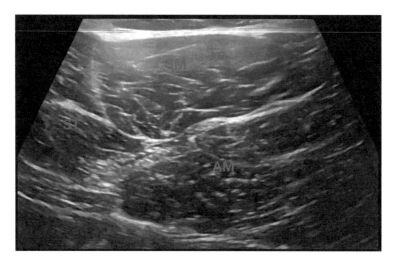

Fig. 14 Transverse view of the hamstring muscles in the mid thigh. ST—semitendinosus. SM—semimembranosus. AM—adductor magnus

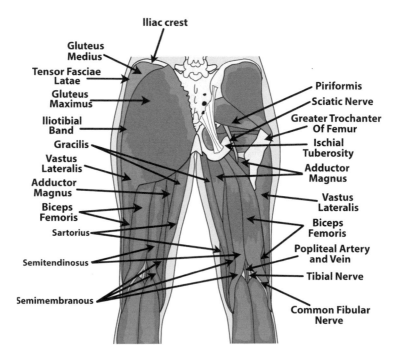

Illustration 3 Illustration highlighting the posterior hip and thigh principal muscles. Figure commissioned by Dr Akram and printed with permission from Unzag Designs

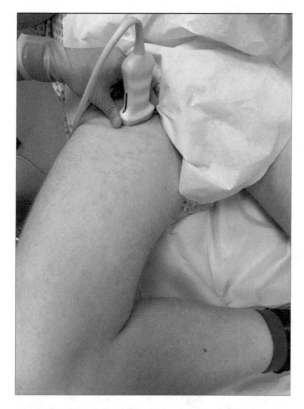

Fig. 15 Longitudinal oblique position of the transducer over the adductor muscles with the hip abducted and knee flexed

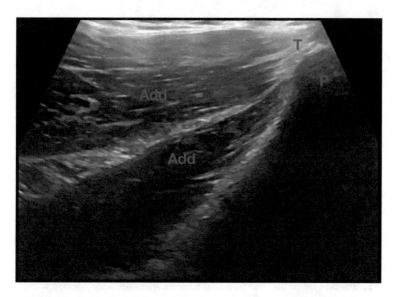

Fig. 16 Longitudinal view of the short adductor muscle group converging onto the pubis. P—pubis. Add—adductor muscles. T—common adductor tendon

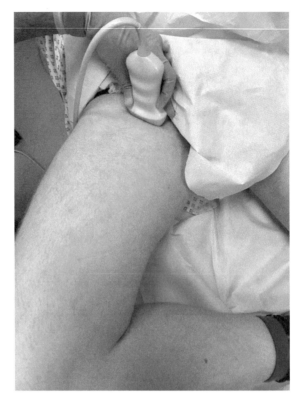

Fig. 17 Transverse position of the transducer over the adductor muscles with the hip abducted and knee flexed

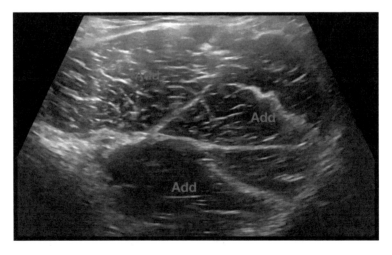

Fig. 18 Transverse view of the short adductors muscles. Add—adductor muscles

Pathology

Ultrasound is a great imaging modality to consider assessment for various hip pathology. As it is a live and dynamic examination, the ultrasound can be used as an extension in the office to complement the clinical history and examination findings, thus help narrow down your differential diagnoses.

Common pathologies encountered include assessment for any underlying joint effusions or synovitis in degenerative or inflammatory arthropathies or even crystal arthritides (Figs. 19, 20, 21, 22). Osseous morphology and detecting enthesophytes can be helpful in the context of diseases. Other common uses include assessment for tendinopathies and concurrent bursitis particularly around the lateral aspect of the hip referring to greater trochanteric pain syndrome (Figs. 23 and 24).

Acknowledgements   Dr Jay Panchal—Musculoskeletal Radiologist.

Mr Niall Rowlands—Reporting Radiographer. Mr Dean Eckersley-Senior Radiographer.

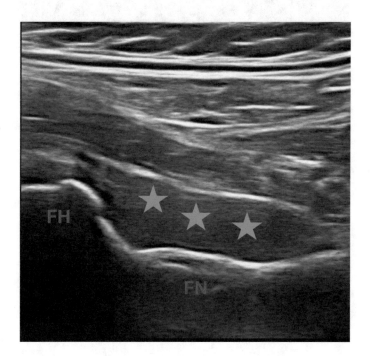

Fig. 19 Longitudinal view of the hip joint. FH—femoral head. FN—femoral neck. *** is synovitis

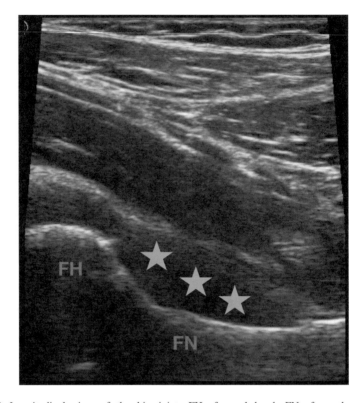

Fig. 20 Longitudinal view of the hip joint. FH—femoral head. FN—femoral neck. ***
is synovitis

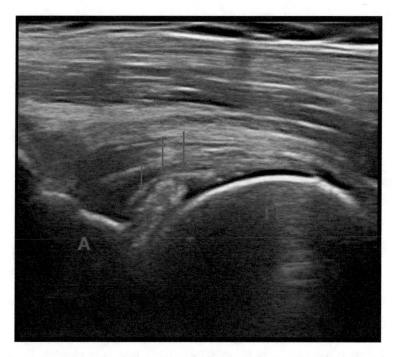

Fig. 21 Longitudinal view of the hip joint. FH—femoral head. A—acetabulum. Red arrows indicate pseudogout

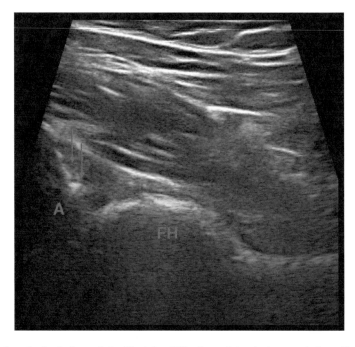

Fig. 22 Longitudinal view of the hip joint. FH—femoral head. A—acetabulum. Red arrows outline osteoarthritis of the joint

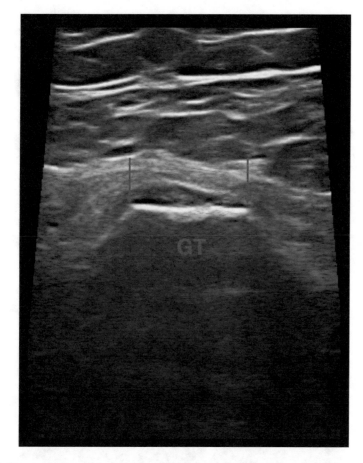

Fig. 23 Transverse view of the lateral hip. Red arrows indicate enthesophytes. GT—greater trochanter

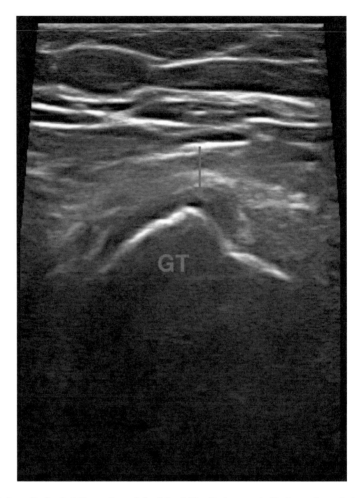

Fig. 24 Longitudinal oblique view of the lateral hip. Red arrow indicates enthesophytes. GT—greater trochanter

References

1. Moller I, Janta I, Backhaus M, et al. The 2017 EULAR standardized procedures for ultrasound imaging in rheumatology. Ann Rheum Dis. 2017;76(12):1974–9.
2. Lin YT, Wang TG. Ultrasonogaphic examination of the adult hip. J Med Ultras. 2012;20(4):201–9.
3. Dawes A, Seidenberg PH. Sonography of sports injuries of the hip. Sports Health. 2014;6(6):531–8.

The Knee Joint

Stuart Wildman

Basic Anatomy

The tibiofemoral joint is formed by the union of the distal femur and proximal tibia. The joint is stabilised by the joint capsule, the medial and lateral collateral ligaments and the anterior and posterior cruciate ligaments. The primary movements performed at the tibiofemoral joint are flexion and extension. The muscles that are evaluated in this region include the quadriceps. Ultrasound can visualise the extensor mechanism including the quadriceps and patella tendon (Illustrations 1 and 2). Posteriorly, the distal hamstring insertions can be seen, along with the division of the sciatic nerve into the tibial and common peroneal nerves.

The articular joint capsule consists of a thin, but strong fibrous membrane which is strengthened almost throughout by other structures supporting it.

Ultrasound Examination Technique

The Suprapatellar Recess and Quadriceps Tendon

To start the examination of the knee joint, the suprapatellar recess and quadricep tendon is evaluated. The patient is positioned in a supine position with the knee at approximately 40° flexion. The probe should be placed in a longitudinal plane (Fig. 1) and the suprapatellar recess and quadriceps tendon will be visualised (Fig. 2). Ensuring the knee is in a flexed position will help avoid anisotropy. The

S. Wildman (✉)
Advanced Practice Physiotherapist and Consultant Musculoskeletal Sonographer,
The Homerton University Hospital NHS Foundation Trust and The Royal Surrey NHS
Foundation Trust, London, UK
e-mail: stuart.wildman1@nhs.uk

Q. Akram and S. Basu (eds.), *Ultrasound in Rheumatology*,
https://doi.org/10.1007/978-3-030-68659-8_6

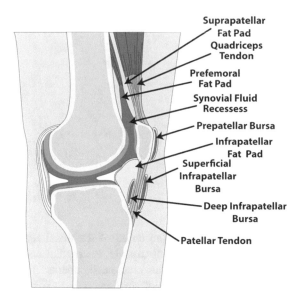

Illustration 1 The anterior knee (Sagittal): This illustration from a sagittal plane correlates with the orientation that is encountered when performing a longitudinal view of the anterior knee structures on ultrasound. This will be viewed initially when interrogating the suprapatellar recess for an effusion, and the extensor mechanism. A number of bursae can also be seen including the pre patellar bursa, deep infrapatellar bursa and superficial infrapatellar bursa in this view. Figure commissioned by Dr Akram and printed with permission from Unzag Designs

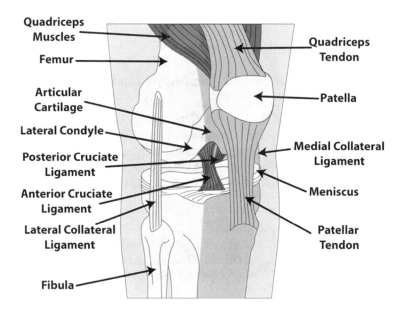

Illustration 2 The anterior knee (coronal): This illustration clearly demonstrates the width of the quadricep and patella tendons, highlighting the importance of moving the transducer throughout the tendon width to ensure pathology is not missed. Often the patella tendon can be at least the width of a linear probe. Figure commissioned by Dr Akram and printed with permission from Unzag Designs

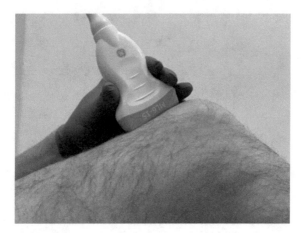

Fig. 1 Patient position and probe position (starting point) for the longitudinal evaluation of the quadriceps tendon and supra-patellar recess. The distal end of the probe is placed on the proximal aspect of the patella. The probe is swept from distal to proximal and medial to lateral to ensure the full length and diameter of the quadriceps tendon is seen and any effusion in the recess is evaluated

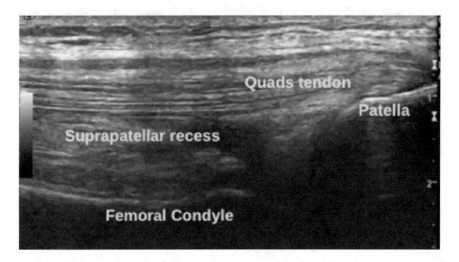

Fig. 2 Longitudinal view of the supra-patellar recess and quadriceps tendon

probe should be moved from lateral to medial to evaluate the suprapatellar recess noting the amount of effusion in comparison to the asymptomatic side, the degree of synovial thickening and the presence of any hyperaemia with power doppler if present [2]. Ensure probe pressure is alternated to avoid compression of collections of joint effusion and synovial thickening.

When evaluating the quadriceps tendon ensure that both the medial insertion of the vastus medialis, the central insertion of the rectus femoris and vastus

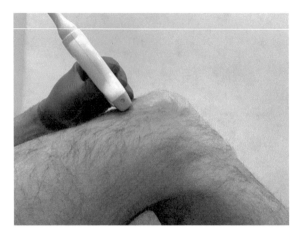

Fig. 3 Patient position and probe position for the transverse evaluation of the quadriceps tendon and articular cartilage. The probe is swept from medial to lateral to ensure both tendon and cartilage seen. To get a better view of the articular cartilage on the femoral condyles, full flexion of the knee is performed

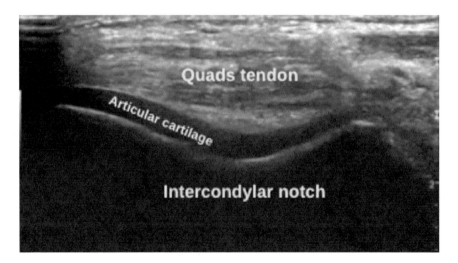

Fig. 4 Transverse view of the quadriceps tendon and articular cartilage. Note the intercondylar notch of the femur

intermedius and the lateral insertion of the vastus lateralis are visualised. This region can also be visualised in a short axis plane (Fig. 3) highlighting the inter-condylar notch of the femur, articular cartilage and joint effusion. The quadriceps tendon can also be visualised in the short axis view, identifying the different lami-nar for each quadricep muscle tendons (Fig. 4). With full flexion of the knee and in short axis an evaluation of the articular cartilage can also be made.

The Patella Tendon (and Infrapatellar Recess)

To visualise the patella tendon the patient should be lying supine with the knee flexed at approximately 30–40°. This ensures the patella tendon is under tension and is therefore easier to visualise with ultrasound.

Place the probe on the distal aspect of the patella directed towards the tibial tuberosity (Fig. 5). Visualise the tendon in a longitudinal view ensuring both the proximal origin from the patella and the distal insertion to the tibial tuberosity are interrogated (Fig. 6) by sweeping the probe from proximal to distal. Evaluate these bony insertions for enthesophytes and erosive change. Doppler can be utilised to evaluate the tendon for hyperaemia and especially at the distal (insertional) enthesis. Ensure probe pressure is light to visualise both the distal superficial, deep infrapatellar bursa and infra-patellar recess.

The tendon can be then be visualised in short axis. Keep the patient in the same position in supine with the knee flexed at 30–40°. Place the probe in a short axis position on the patella tendon (Fig. 7). The patella tendon will be seen as a hyperechoic structure (Fig. 8). Note that the patella tendon can sometimes be wider than the width of a linear probe and therefore moving fully from lateral to medial is required.

Medial Parapatellar Recess

To visualise the medial parapatellar recess the patient should be positioned in supine with the knee in a relaxed and extended position (Fig. 9). The ultrasound

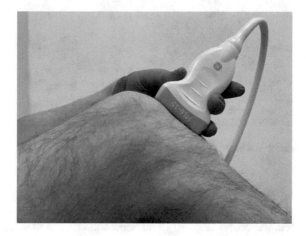

Fig. 5 Patient position and probe position of the patella tendon. The probe is swept from proximal to distal and medial to lateral. The pre-patellar and infra-patellar bursa can be identified at this level

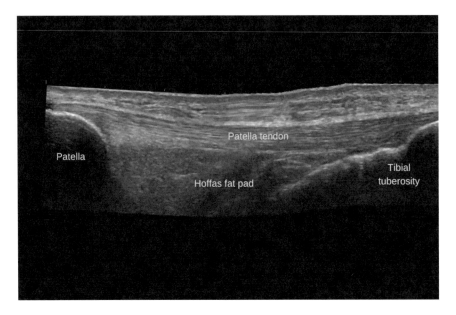

Fig. 6 Longitudinal panoramic view of the patella tendon

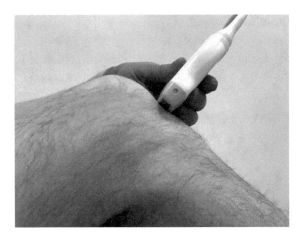

Fig. 7 Patient position and probe position for the transverse view of the patella tendon

probe should be placed on the medial border of the patella angled towards the medial joint line. The medial patellar retinaculum can be visualised along with the medial patellofemoral recess (Fig. 10). This view can be used to visualise an effusion and synovial thickening.

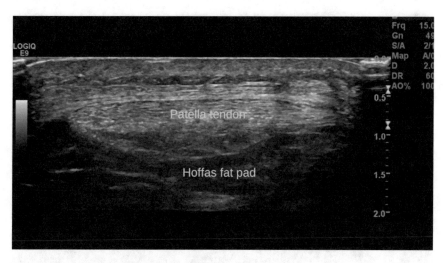

Fig. 8 Transverse scan of the patellar tendon

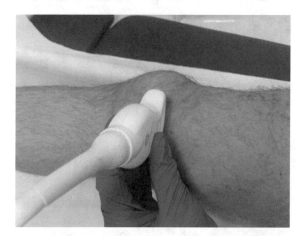

Fig. 9 Patient position and probe position of the medial parapatellar recess. The proximal end of the probe is placed on the femoral condyle and the distal end of the probe on the patella

The Medial Knee

To visualise the medial joint line of the tibiofemoral joint the patient should be positioned in supine with the knee extended (Fig. 11). If the leg is externally rotated it also facilitates visualisation of this region. Ensure there is a clear understanding of the proximal and distal aspects of the ultrasound image. It is then

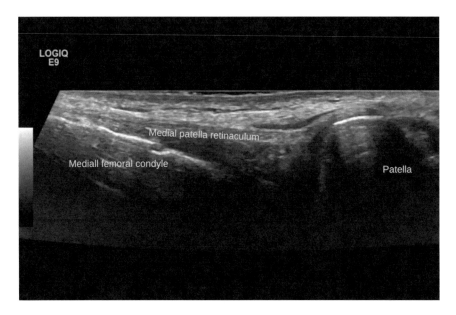

Fig. 10 Longitudinal view of the medial parapatellar recess and retinaculum

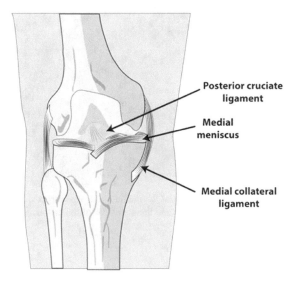

Illustration 3 The medial knee (coronal): This illustration highlights the position of the medial collateral ligament. Often it can be easier to identify by highlighting it at its femoral origin and then moving the probe distally. Figure commissioned by Dr Akram and printed with permission from Unzag Designs

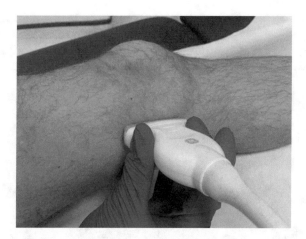

Fig. 11 Patient position and probe position of the medial tibio-femoral joint. The proximal probe is placed on the medial femoral condyle and the distal aspect on the medial tibial condyle. The medial collateral ligament and medial mensici can also be seen at this level. Note this is the left leg

possible to visualise the medial joint recess of the tibiofemoral joint (Fig. 12) evaluating for joint narrowing and bony hypertrophy. The deep and superficial medial collateral ligament can also be seen superficial to the joint line.

Pes Anserine

To visualise the pes anserine tendons, visualise the tibiofemoral joint and move the probe distal and angled medially to the tibial shaft. (Fig. 13). The Pes Anserine tendons of Sartorius, Gracilis and Semitendinosus can be seen to insert to the shaft of the tibia (Fig. 14).

Lateral Parapatellar Recess

To visualise the lateral parapatellar recess the patient should be positioned in supine with the knee in a relaxed and extended position. The ultrasound probe should be placed on the lateral border of the patella angled towards the lateral joint line (Fig. 15). The lateral patellar retinaculum can be visualised along with the lateral patellofemoral recess (Fig. 16).

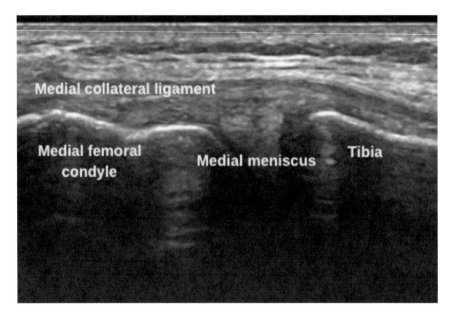

Fig. 12 Longitudinal scan of the tibio-femoral joint medial including the medial collateral ligament and the menisci

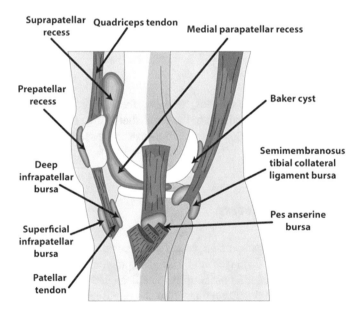

Illustration 4 Pes anserine (sagittal): The pes anserine tendon can be clearly visualised on ultrasound but it is often difficult to differentiate between the three tendons of the gracilis, semintendinous and sartorius. Figure commissioned by Dr Akram and printed with permission from Unzag Designs

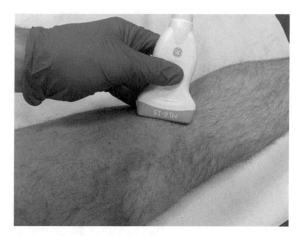

Fig. 13 Patient position and probe position of the pes anserine complex. The probe is longitudinal to the tibia and transverse to the pes anserine tendons

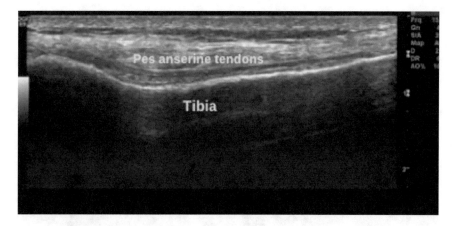

Fig. 14 Longitudinal view of the Pes Anserine complex (sartorius, gracilis, semitendinosus)

The Lateral Knee

To visualise the lateral joint line of the tibiofemoral joint the patient should be positioned in supine with the knee extended (Fig. 17). It is also possible to visualise this region with the patient in side lying. Ensure there is a clear understanding of the proximal and distal aspects of the image. It is important to visualise the lateral joint recess of the tibiofemoral joint evaluating for joint narrowing and bony hypertrophy, and also the popliteal tendon (Fig. 18). The ITB can be seen clearly to insert to the Gerdy's tubercle on the tibia (Fig. 19). The lateral collateral

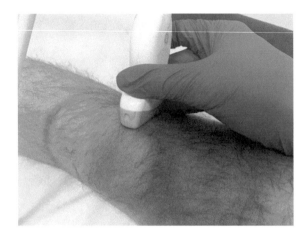

Fig. 15 Patient position and probe position for examination lateral parapatellar recess. The proximal end of the probe is on the lateral femoral condyle and the distal aspect on the patella. Note: this is an examination of a right leg

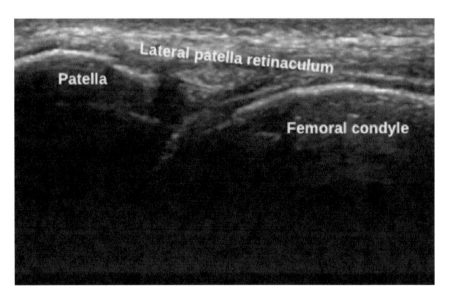

Fig. 16 Longitudinal view of the lateral parapatellar recess and retinaculum

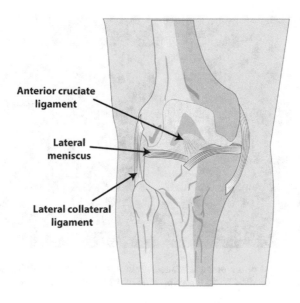

Illustration 5 The lateral knee (coronal): This illustration highlights the lateral meniscus in the lateral aspect of the tibiofemoral joint. The lateral collateral ligament can be seen superficial to this inserting distally to the fibular head. Knowledge of bony landmarks is key to enable accurate sonographic identification of structures in this region. Figure commissioned by Dr Akram and printed with permission from Unzag Designs

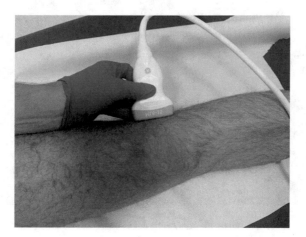

Fig. 17 Patient position and probe position of the lateral knee joint. The proximal probe is on the lateral femoral condyle and the distal probe on the fibula head. The lateral tibiofemoral joint line can be viewed at this level. Note: this is left leg of patient

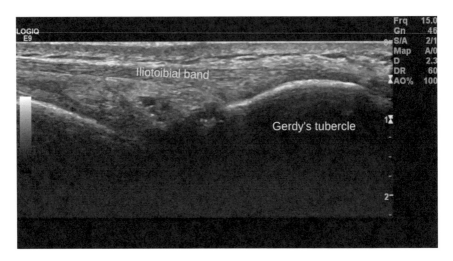

Fig. 18 The distal end of the probe is rotated slightly medially to the gerdy's tubercle on the tibia to view the characteristic broad distal insertion of the Iliotibial band (ITB)

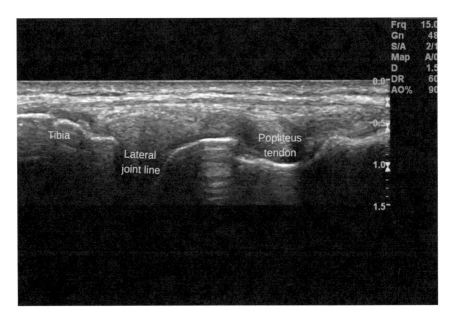

Fig. 19 The lateral aspect of the tibiofemoral joint is visualised between the tibia and femoral condyle. The location of the popliteal tendon can also be seen

ligament can also be seen attaching to the fibula head (Fig. 20). This structure can often be difficult to visualise in its entirety due to its length but also to the wavy nature of it when not under tension.

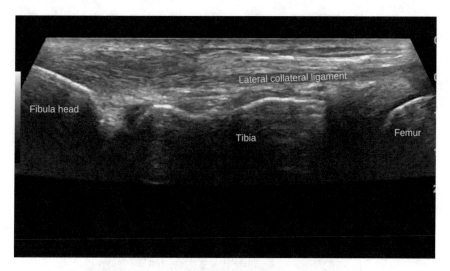

Fig. 20 Longitudinal view of the lateral collateral ligament inserting to the fibula head

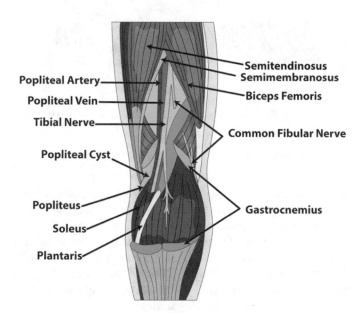

Illustration 6 The posterior knee (coronal): Evaluating this region on ultrasound requires excellent knowledge of the musculature in this region including the gastrocnemius and the distal hamstring tendons. Centrally located, the sciatic nerve will also be seen prior to it dividing into the tibial and common peroneal (fibular) branches. Figure commissioned by Dr Akram and printed with permission from Unzag Designs

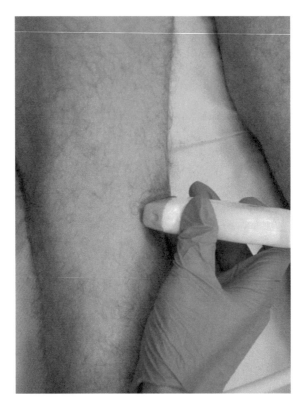

Fig. 21 Patient position and probe position posteromedial knee joint. One end of the probe is placed on the medial femoral condyle and the other over the medial head of gastrocnemius and semi-membranous tendon. Probe should be swept from medial to lateral and proximal to distal

The Posterior Knee

To visualise the posteromedial aspect of the knee joint, position the patient in prone lying with the knee in full extension (Fig. 21). If the patient is unable to fully extend the knee, then place a pillow under the ankle as this can help the patient feel more comfortable. Place the probe on the posteromedial aspect of the knee in a short axis view (Fig. 22). It is possible to visualise the small and very superficial tendon of the semitendinosus (ST), and deep to this the semimembranosus tendon (SM). Medial to this is the prominent bony outline of the medial femoral condyle. Lateral to the hamstring tendons the medial gastrocnemius muscle can be seen to provide a lateral border. Baker's cysts will commonly appear in the fascial plane between the semitendinosus and semimembranosus tendons and the medial head of gastrocnemius.

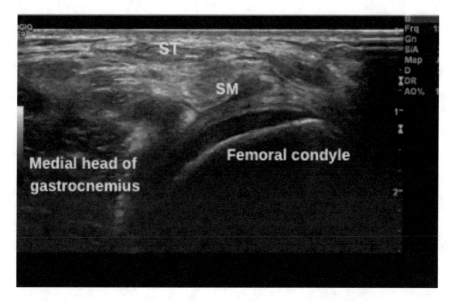

Fig. 22 Transverse view of the posteromedial knee. SM- semimembranous and ST- semitendinosus tendon. The region between these two structures is where a Bakers cyst would be visualised (See Fig. 26)

Pathology

The evaluation of the supra-patellar, medial and lateral recesses as well as the infra-patellar recess can identify effusions or presence of synovitis/synovial hypertrophy (Figs. 23, 24). Synovial hypertrophy is abnormal, hypoechoic tissue that is non-displaceable and poorly compressible [3]. It is important to acknowledge the prevalence of synovial effusions and hypertrophy in normal joints such as metatarsophalangeal joints of the feet, in particular the 1st MTPJ [6]. A clinician's appreciation of what is 'normal' is often a key foundation of appropriate ultrasound use [4, 5].

There may also be co-existing doppler signal, however this can be more difficult to interpret due to the tissue depth of the knee in comparison to more superficial joints such as the metacarpophalangeal joints in the hand. The impact of using different machines, doppler modalities and settings has also been shown to have a considerable impact on the quantification of inflammation [6].

Knee joint effusions are easily evaluated on ultrasound and better than a clinical examination [4, 5]. Comparison between asymptomatic and symptomatic joints can often provide useful clinical information.

Joint effusions associated with osteoarthritis and inflammatory arthritis can often lead to a Bakers cyst, that can be seen in the posteromedial aspect of the knee (Fig. 25).

Osteoarthritis causes characteristic osteophytes which can be seen at the joint margins of the tibiofemoral joint (Fig. 26). Menisci can also be extruded. Cartilage

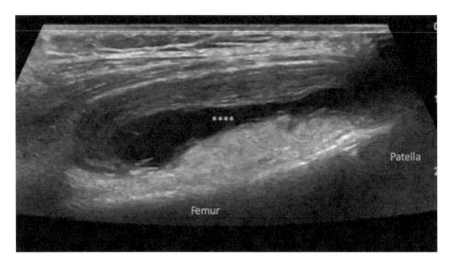

Fig. 23 Longitudinal view of supra-patellar recess and synovitis. **** indicates synovitis

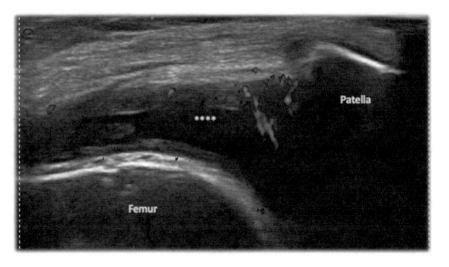

Fig. 24 Longitudinal view of the lateral parapatellar recess showing synovitis (****) with doppler activity

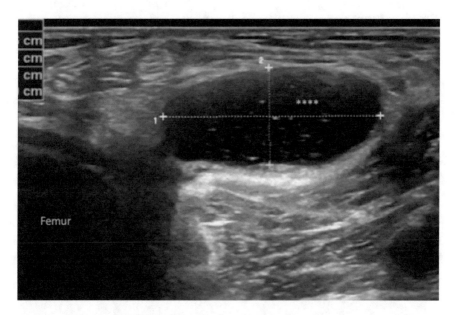

Fig. 25 Transverse scan of the posterior knee showing Baker's cyst (****)

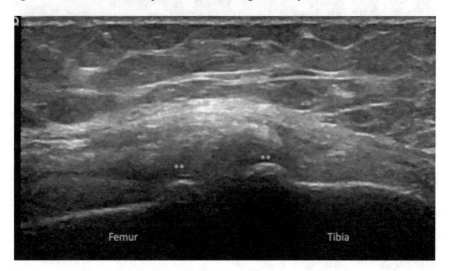

Fig. 26 Longitudinal view of lateral knee showing osteophytes (**)

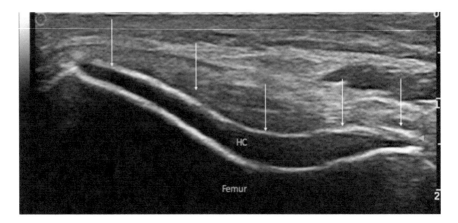

Fig. 27 Transverse view of the articular cartilage showing double contour sign (white arrows) in gout

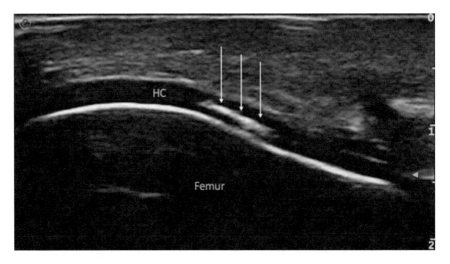

Fig. 28 Transverse view of the articular cartilage showing crystal deposition within articular cartilage (white arrows) in pseudo-gout

thinning can also be seen at the level of the femoral condyle. When evaluating the cartilage at the level of the femoral condyle a double contour sign is seen in gout [7] (Fig. 27) and deposition of crystal within the cartilage indicates pseudo-gout or CPPD (Fig. 28). Other features can include gouty tophi (Fig. 29) and crystal deposits in the menisci.

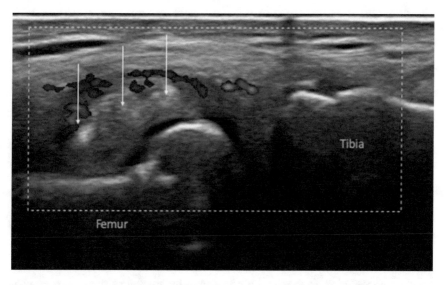

Fig. 29 Longitudinal view of tibio-femoral joint demonstrating gout tophi (white arrows). Doppler activity surrounding the tophi

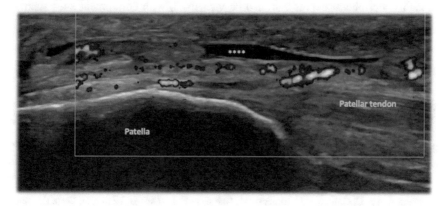

Fig. 30 Longitudinal view of the patellar tendon showing a pre-patellar bursitis with doppler activity (****)

There are many bursae around the knee including the prepatellar and deep infrapatellar bursae (Fig. 30). Bursae are extra-articular structures that reduce friction [8]. Sonographic pathological changes may include being distended, with either a hypoechoic or anechoic appearance and positive doppler signal.

Spondyloarthopathies can cause enthesitis and typically this can be seen at the insertion sites of the quadriceps and patella tendon (Fig. 31). Enthesitis often occurs at the fibrocartilaginous entheses [9]. Differentiating mechanical insertional

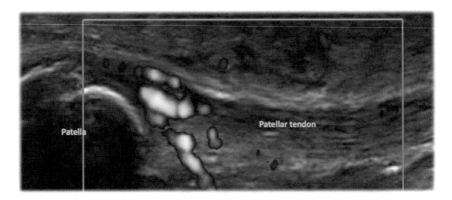

Fig. 31 Longitudinal view of the patellar tendon demonstrating doppler activity at the superior portion of the patella tendon seen in spondyloarthopathies

tendon complaints from those with a systemic inflammatory driver can be challenging and utilising ultrasound can be helpful.

Ultrasound is able to evaluate acute muscle, tendon and ligament injuries in this region, although not intraarticular injuries where MRI is the choice of imaging modality. Peripheral nerves can also be visualised, with entrapment sites such as the common peroneal nerve at the fibula head being easily accessible.

References

1. Wakefield RJ, Balint PV, Szkudlarek M, Filippucci E, Backhaus M, D'Agostino MA, Sanchez EN, Iagnocco A, Schmidt WA, Bruyn GA, Bruyn G. Musculoskeletal ultrasound including definitions for ultrasonographicpathology. J Rheumatology. 2005;32(12):2485–7.
2. D'Agostino MA, Terslev L, Aegerter P, Backhaus M, Balint P, Bruyn GA, Filippucci E, Grassi W, Iagnocco A, Jousse-Joulin S, Kane D. Scoring ultrasound synovitis in rheumatoid arthritis: a EULAR-OMERACT ultrasound taskforce—Part 1: definition and development of a standardised, consensus-based scoring system. RMD Open. 2017;3(1):e000428.
3. Najm A, Orr C, Gallagher L, Biniecka M, Gaigneux E, Le Goff B, Fearon U, Veale DJ. Knee joint synovitis: study of correlations and diagnostic performances of ultrasonography compared with histopathology. RMD Open, 2018;4(1).
4. Kane D, Balint PV, Sturrock RD. Ultrasonography is superior to clinical examination in the detection and localization of knee joint effusion in rheumatoid arthritis. J Rheumatol. 2003;30(5):966–71.
5. Padovano I, Costantino F, Breban M, D'agostino MA. Prevalence of ultrasound synovial inflammatory findings in healthy subjects. Annals Rheum Diseas. 2016;75(10):1819–23.
6. Torp-Pedersen S, Christensen R, Szkudlarek M, Ellegaard K, D'Agostino MA, Iagnocco A, Naredo E, Balint P, Wakefield RJ, Torp-Pedersen A, Terslev L. Power and color Doppler ultrasound settings for inflammatory flow: impact on scoring of disease activity in patients with rheumatoid arthritis. Arthrit Rheumatol. 2015;67(2):386–95.

7. Bhadu D, Das SK, Wakhlu A, Dhakad U, Sharma M. Ultrasonographic detection of double contour sign and hyperechoic aggregates for diagnosis of gout: two sites examination is as good as six sites examination. Int J Rheum Diseas. 2018;21(2):523–31.
8. Ruangchaijatuporn T, Gaetke-Udager K, Jacobson JA, Yablon CM, Morag Y. Ultrasound evaluation of bursae: anatomy and pathological appearances. Skeletal Radiol. 2017;46(4):445–62.
9. Kaeley GS, Eder L, Aydin SZ, Gutierrez M, Bakewell C. Enthesitis: a hallmark of psoriatic arthritis. In: Seminars in arthritis and rheumatism, vol. 48, no. 1. WB Saunders; 2018. pp. 35–43.

The Ankle and Foot

Qasim Akram

Ankle Examination

Anterior Ankle

Basic Anatomy

The ankle is a hinge joint. It arises due to a mortice formed by the lateral malleoli (of the fibula) and the lower end of the tibia and body of the talus (tibiotalar joint). The capsule of the joint fits closely around its articular surfaces and as in every hinge joint it is weak anteriorly and posteriorly but reinforced laterally and medially by strong collateral ligaments (Illustration 1) [1].

The ankle joint can be flexed (plantar flexion) and extended (dorsiflexion). The main dorsiflexors are tibialis anterior, extensor digitorum longus and extensor hallucis longus which are seen anteriorly (Illustration 2). The principal plantar flexors are tibialis posterior, flexor hallucis longus and flexor digitorum longus which are seen medially (Illustration 3). The lateral tendons include the peroneus brevis and longus tendons (Illustration 4). Inversion is created by the anterior and medial tendons whereas the lateral tendons cause eversion. The midtarsal joints allow gliding movements of the entire foot [2].

The tibialis anterior courses the anterior aspect of the ankle lateral to medial cuneiform and plantar aspect of base of the first metatarsal. The extensor hallucis lies between tibialis anterior and the extensor digitorum longus tendons being lateral to the former and medial to latter. The extensor digitorum longus passes over anterior ankle and inserts on the middle and distal phalanges of the second through fifth toes (Illustration 2) [3].

Q. Akram (✉)
Stockport NHS Foundation Trust, Stockport, UK
e-mail: qasim.akram.qa@gmail.com

© The Author(s), under exclusive license to Springer Nature Switzerland AG 2021   157
Q. Akram and S. Basu (eds.), *Ultrasound in Rheumatology*,
https://doi.org/10.1007/978-3-030-68659-8_7

The subtalar joint is formed by the articulation of the talus and calcaneum (Illustrations 5, 6). It is supported by a fibrous capsule which is attached to the margins of the articular facets and reinforced by the talocalcaneal ligaments. The anterior subtalar joint lies where head of talus articulates with the posterior surface of navicular bone, the superior aspect of the spring ligament, sustentacular tali (of the calcaneum) and the articular surface of the calcaneus [2, 3].

The foot can be subdivided into three parts: the hindfoot (talus, calcaneus), the midfoot (navicular, cuboid, and 3 cuneiforms) and the forefoot (metatarsals (MT), phalanges) (Illustrations 1, 7).

Bones of the ankle and foot include calcaneum, talus, navicular, cuboid (articulates with 4th and 5th metatarsals), cuneiforms (lateral, intermediate, medial) and articulate with 1-3rd metatarsals. There are 5 metatarsals and 5 phalanges containing distal, intermediate and proximal phalanges. The great toe metatarso-phalanx (MTP) only has a proximal and a distal phalanx [2, 3].

The transverse tarsal joint, consisting of the talonavicular joint medially and the calcaneocuboid joint (Illustration 7) laterally allows inversion and eversion. In a more distal location, the navicular articulates with the 3 cuneiforms. The cuneiforms and cuboid articulate with base of the 5 metatarsals forming the tarsometatarsal joints [3].

More distally, the forefoot joints MTPJs, proximal and distal IP joints allow graded flexion and extension of the great toe and the lesser toes (Illustration 7) [3].

A linear probe is usually used for the ankle and foot (8-15 MHz) but a higher frequency probe (such as hockey stick can be used) mainly for the smaller and more peripheral joints of the foot. Please ensure that adequate depth and focus is used. One hand should be used to control the US machine and its settings and the other to scan the relevant joint area [4, 5].

To start the examination of the ankle joint the tibiotalar joint and anterior recess are evaluated. The patient is asked to lie in a supine position with flexion of the knees and the foot being placed flat on the examination couch. The probe is placed in the midline of the ankle to obtain a longitudinal (or long axis) view of the tibio-talar joint (Figs. 1, 2). The probe is swept from proximal to distal to evaluate the anterior recess of the tibiotalar joint for any excess synovial fluid. The probe is then placed in a transverse view through a 180-degree swivel and on this view the integrity of the hyaline articular cartilage can be made [4, 5].

The probe is then swept further distally in a longitudinal view and in line or parallel to the 2nd metatarsal bone to identify **the talonavicular, naviculo-cuneiform and then the tarso(cuneiform)metatarsal joints** (Figs. 3, 4, 5). The 3 cuneiform bones and joints can be viewed in a transverse view (Figs. 6, 7). The middle cuneiform articulates with the 2nd metatarsal head [4].

The patient is placed in the same position and an examination of the anterior extensor tendons is made. The probe is placed in transverse view first and swept from medial to lateral (Figs. 8, 9) to examine each of the 3 anterior extensor tendons. Then each individual tendon is seen in longitudinal view sweeping the probe from proximal to distal (Figs. 10, 11) [4].

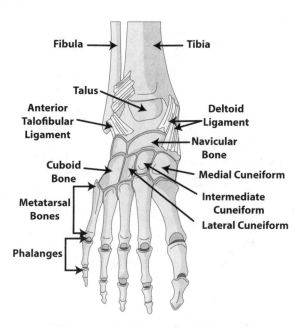

Illustration 1 Illustration of the anterior ankle including tibio-talar joint, mid-tarsal and inter-phalangeal joints. Figure commissioned by Dr Akram and printed with permission from Unzag Designs

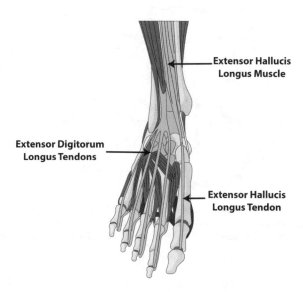

Illustration 2 Illustration of the anterior extensor tendons including extensor hallucis longus and extensor digitorum longus tendons. Tibialis anterior is located medial to the extensor hallucis tendon and is a dorsiflexor. This is better shown on Illustration 4. Figure commissioned by Dr Akram and printed with permission from Unzag Designs

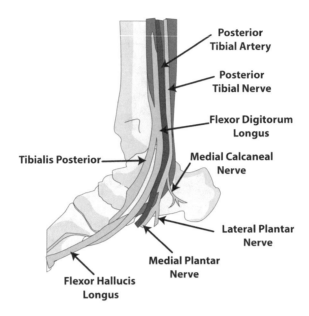

Illustration 3 Illustration of the medial flexor tendons- tibialis posterior, flexor digitorum longus and then fleor hallucis longus. Figure commissioned by Dr Akram and printed with permission from Unzag Designs

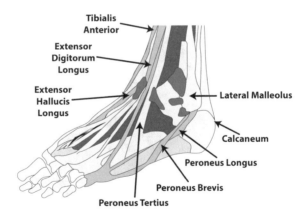

Illustration 4 Anatomical diagram of lateral tendons- peroneal longus and brevis. On this you can see the anterior tendons- lateral to medial- extensor digitorum, extensor hallucis longus and tibialis anterior. Figure commissioned by Dr Akram and printed with permission from Unzag Designs

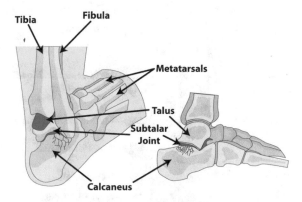

Illustration 5 Diagram of the sub-talar joint. Figure commissioned by Dr Akram and printed with permission from Unzag Designs

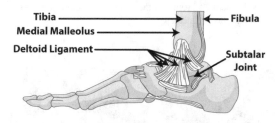

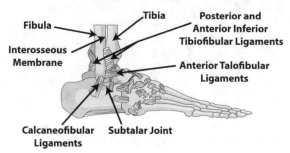

Illustration 6 Lateral and medial view of ankle joint including medial deltoid ligaments and then lateral tibio-fibular, talo-fibular and calcaneo-fibular ligaments. Figure commissioned by Dr Akram and printed with permission from Unzag Designs

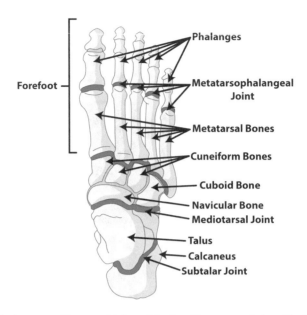

Illustration 7   Anatomy of bones and joints of the foot. Figure commissioned by Dr Akram and printed with permission from Unzag Designs

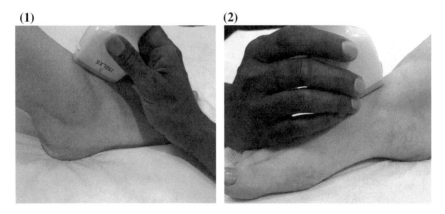

Fig. 1   Patient position and probe position (starting point) for the longitudinal evaluation of tibio-totalar joint and anterior recess (1.1) and them midtarsal joints (1.2)

To examine **the anterior tibio-fibular ligament** (Illustration 6) one end of the probe is placed on the lateral malleoli(fibula) and the other end rotated in a slightly oblique position and towards the the distal tibia. The distal tibia and lateral malleolus(fibula) should be seen on the sonoanatomy image (Figs. 12, 13).

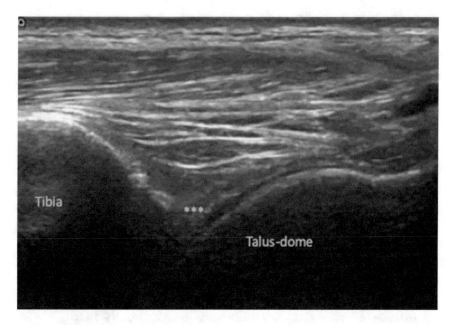

Fig. 2 Longitudinal scan of the anterior ankle. Tibiotalar joint and anterior recess. *** represents anterior recess

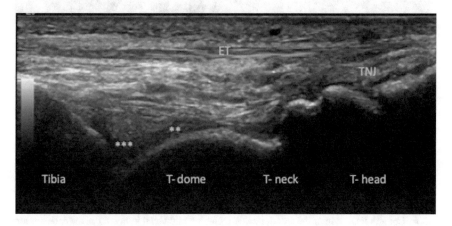

Fig. 3 Longitudinal scan of the anterior ankle including mid tarsal joints. ET is the extensor tendon. TNJ is the talo-navicular joint. T is Talus. ** is the cartilage and *** is the anterior recess

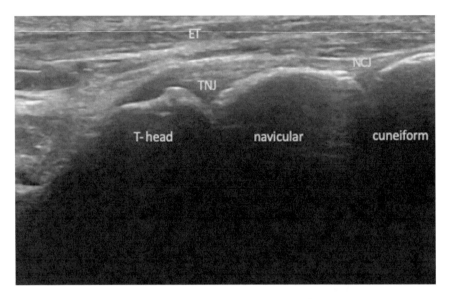

Fig. 4 Longitudinal scan of the anterior ankle including mid tarsal joints. ET is the extensor tendon. TNJ is the talo-navicular joint. NCJ is the naviculo-cuneiform joint. T is Talus

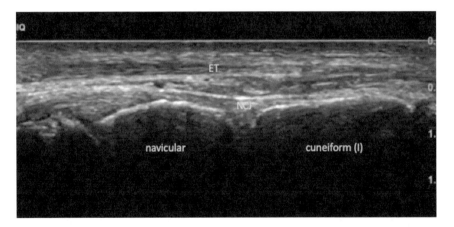

Fig. 5 Longitudinal scan of the anterior ankle including mid tarsal joints. ET is the extensor tendon. NCJ is the naviculo-cuneiform joint

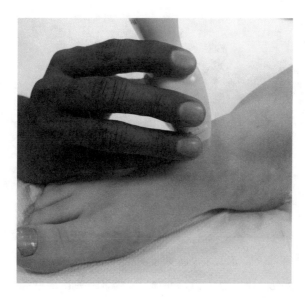

Fig. 6 Patient position and probe position (starting point) for the transverse evaluation of the cuneiform bones

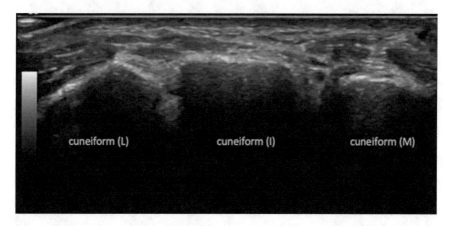

Fig. 7 Transverse scan of the cuneiform bones. L is lateral. I is intermediate and M is medial

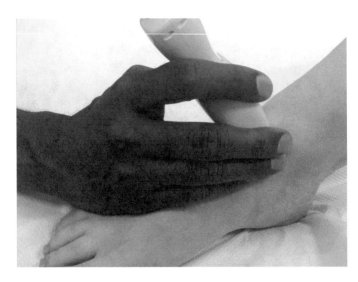

Fig. 8 Patient position and probe position for the transverse evaluation of the anterior extensor tendons

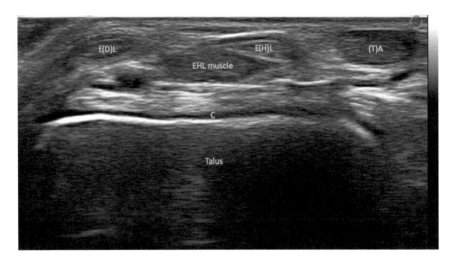

Fig. 9 Transverse scan of the anterior extensor tendons. Medial is Tibialis Anterior, Extensor Digitorum and Extensor Hallucis longus tendon. C is cartilage. T is talus

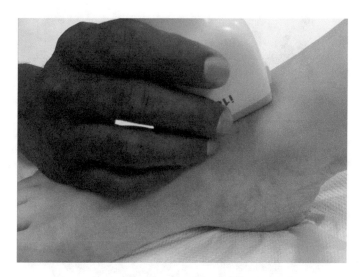

Fig. 10 Patient position and probe position for the longitudinal evaluation of the anterior tendons

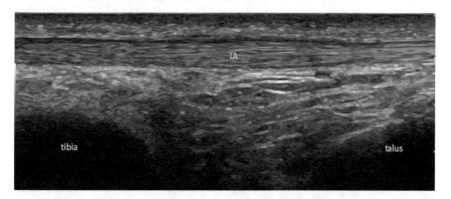

Fig. 11 Longitudinal view of the (TA) Tibialis Anterior tendon

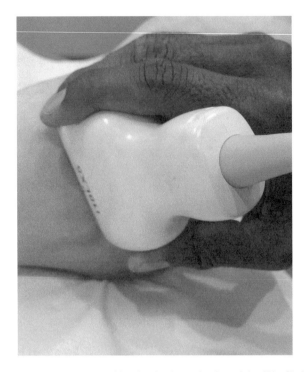

Fig. 12 Patient position and probe position for the the evaluation of the tibio-fibular ligament

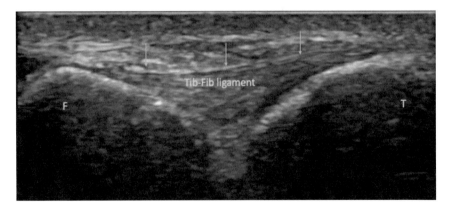

Fig. 13 Long axis view of the tibio-fibular ligament. F is fibula and T is Talus

(1)   **(2)**   **(3)**

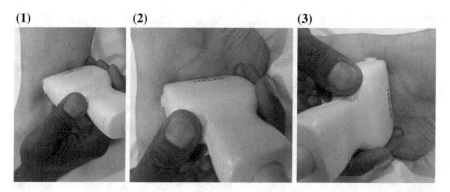

Fig. 14 Patient position and probe position (starting point) for the transverse evaluation of the medial flexor tendons. 14.1 to 14.3 shows the movement of the probe to examine the tendons in medial view

Medial Ankle

Basic Anatomy

The medial tendons consist of three flexor tendons- the tibialis posterior, flexor digitorum longus and flexor hallucis longus- which travels through tarsal tunnel surrounded by separate tendon sheaths. The tibialis posterior is oval in shape and is twice as large as the adjacent flexor digitorum longus. It courses beneath the medial malleolus which it uses as a pulley and superficial to the spring ligament to insert onto the navicular bone sending extensions to the three cuneiforms and bases of first to 4th metatarsals. The tibialis posterior acts as an inverter of the foot and a major stabiliser of the hindfoot. The flexor digitorum longus passes lateral to tibialis posterior and the flexor hallucis is most lateral of the tendons (Illustration 3) [1, 3, 4].

The **tibialis posterior, flexor digitorum longus and flexor hallucis longus (Figs. 14, 15)** are examined with the patient in a similar supine position and knee flexed but this time the hip is abducted to give a good angle to view the medial tendons. The foot can also be everted slightly. The probe is placed in a transverse view just posterior to the distal end of the medial malleolus. The probe is moved from medial to lateral identifying the 3 flexor tendons and the tibial nerve and tarsal tunnel and vessels. Following this, a longitudinal view (Figs. 16, 17) can be obtained of the individual tendons. For example, by placing the probe posterior to

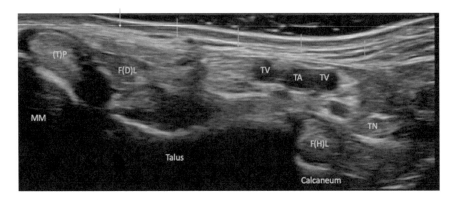

Fig. 15 Transverse evaluation of the flexor tendons. Tibialis Posterior (TP), Flexor Digitorum longus (FDL) and Flexor Hallucis longus (FHL). TA is tibial artery, TV is tibial vein and TN is tibial nerve. MM is medial malleolus

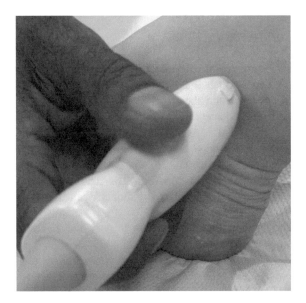

Fig. 16 Patient position and probe position of the longitudinal evaluation of the flexor tendons

the medial malleoli in long axis and then sweeping from proximal to distal including looking at the insertion of the tibialis posterior on the navicular bone (Figs. 18, 19). An easier way to do this, is to actually place the distal end of the probe on the navicular bone and the proximal end of the probe towards the medial malleoli [4].

Following this, the talocalcaneal joint (anterior or medial subtalar joint) is evaluated (Figs. 20, 21) with the patient in the same position looking for any synovial fluid. A long axis view is obtained with sweeping probe from the proximal

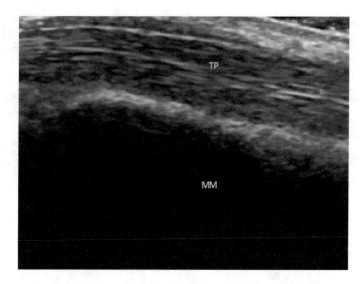

Fig. 17 Longitudinal evaluation of the flexor tendons. TP is Tibialis Posterior. MM is medial malleolus

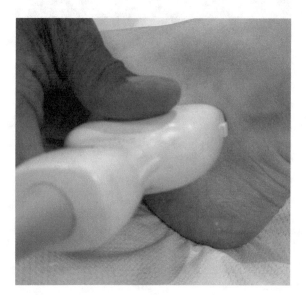

Fig. 18 Patient position and probe position of the longitudinal evaluation of the flexor tendons. Insertion of the tibialis posterior on the navicular bone

sustenaculum tali (of the calcaneum) to the more distal navicular bone. The spring ligament can also be viewed in this position. To look for **the (spring) or calca-neo-navicular ligament (Illustration 6)** the proximal probe is placed on the

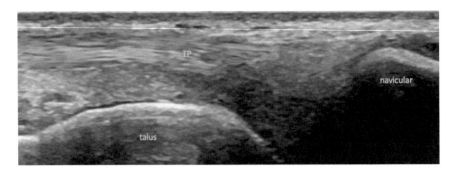

Fig. 19 Longitudinal evaluation of the flexor tendons. Insertion of the tibialis posterior (TP) on the navicular bone

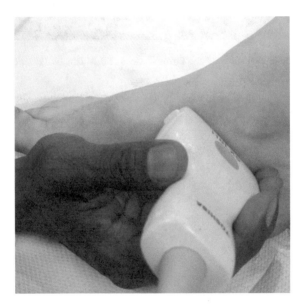

Fig. 20 Patient position and probe position for the longitudinal evaluation of the spring ligament and talo-calcaneal joint (lateral subtalar)

(sustenaculum tali of) calcaneum and distal towards the top of the navicular bone **(Figs. 20, 21)** [4, 5].

The **deltoid ligament (Illustrations 6 and 8) is essentially seen in same position with a slight dorsiflexion of the foot**. Once the tibio-calcaneal joint is seen, move the probe is moved in a fan shaped fashion and in a clockwise direction maintaining one end of the probe on the medial malleoli and the other over the talus, calcaneum and navicular (Figs. 22, 23) [5].

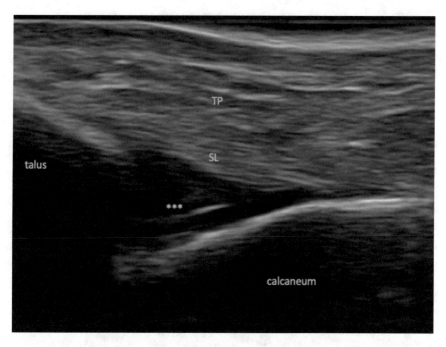

Fig. 21 Longitudinal view of spring ligament. TP is tibialis posterior. SL is spring ligament. *** is the subtalar joint (lateral). Talo-calcaneal joint is long axis

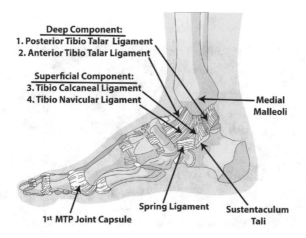

Illustration 8 Illustration of the deltoid ligament. Figure commissioned by Dr Akram and printed with permission from Unzag Designs

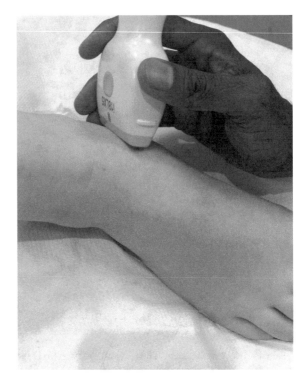

Fig. 22 Patient position and probe position for the longitudinal evaluation of the deltoid ligament

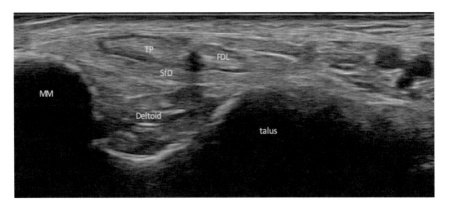

Fig. 23 Longitudinal view of the deltoid ligament. MM is medial malleolus. TP is tibialis posterior. FDL is flexor digitorum longus. SFD is superficial deltoid

Lateral Ankle

Basic Anatomy

The examination of the lateral ankle starts with an examination of the lateral recess of the tibiotalar joint. The patient is placed in a supine position resting on the bed with the knee flexed and plantar aspect of foot on examination table. A slight inversion of the foot can be applied. The US probe is placed at lateral aspect of ankle over lateral malleoli (Figs. 24, 25) [1, 3, 4].

The **posterior or lateral subtalar joint** (Illustration 5) is then examined and can be seen by placing the probe in a longitudinal view as shown. The talus and calcaneum as shown in the sonoanatomy image (Figs. 26, 27) [4, 5].

The lateral tendons are the peroneus longus and peroneus brevis and responsible for eversion of the foot **(Illustration 4)**. These course posterior and inferior to the lateral malleolus which is used as a pulley during contraction of the peroneal muscles. Peroneus brevis is smaller and lies in front of the peroneus longus in the retro malleolar groove on the posterior border of the lateral malleolus. The peroneal brevis is closest to the bone. The peroneus longus passes along the underside of the foot in a groove in the cuboid bone and inserts on lateral side of base of 1st metatarsal and the medial cuneiform [4].

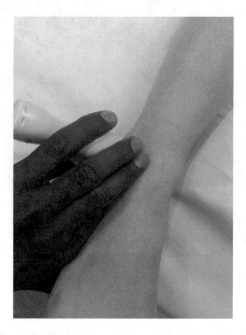

Fig. 24 Patient position and probe position of the longitudinal view of the lateral recess

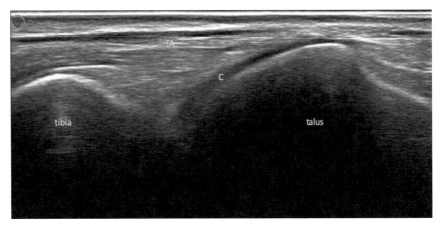

Fig. 25 Longitudinal view of the lateral recess

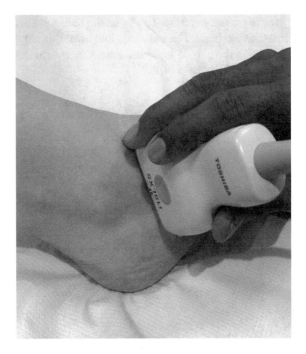

Fig. 26 Patient position and probe position of the longitudinal evaluation of the lateral subtalar joint

To examine these tendons, the patient is placed in the same position as the previous lateral structures and the foot is then inverted slightly, with the. **The peroneal tendons can then be seen** by placing the US probe posterior to the lateral malleolus and over the retro-fibular groove. Initially, a transverse view is obtained,

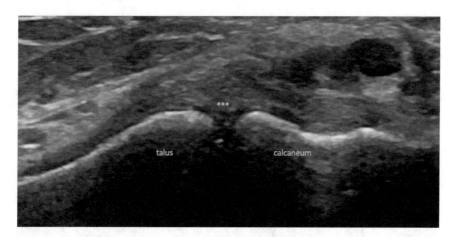

Fig. 27 Longitudinal view of subtalar (lateral) joint

(1)   **(2)**

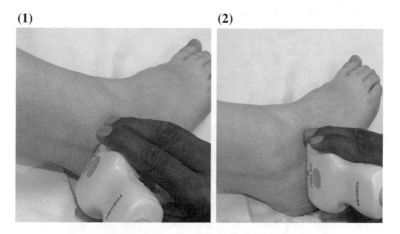

Fig. 28 Patient position and probe position for the transverse evaluation of the peroneal tendons. 28.1 and 28.2 show the direction of the probe movement in capturing these tendons

and the probe is swept from medial to lateral (Figs. 28, 29). In longitudinal view, the probe is swept from proximal to distal (Figs. 30, 31) all the way down to the insertion of the peroneal brevis tendon on the 5th MTP (Figs. 32, 33) [4].

In this same position, the **anterior talo-fibular ligament (ATFL) (Illustrations 6 and 9)** is examined. A slightly inverted foot position will stretch the lateral ligaments. The probe is placed longitudinally from the lateral malleolus(fibula) to the talus and almost being parallel to the sole of foot. The lateral malleoli and talus are seen in the sonoanatomy image (Figs. 34, 35) [3, 4].

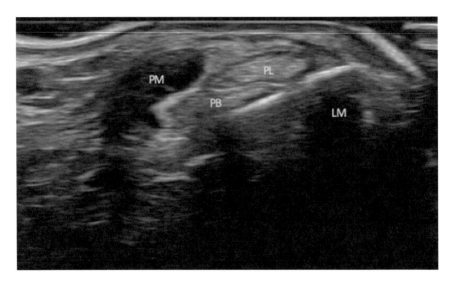

Fig. 29 Transverse scan of the peroneal tendons. PL is peroneal longus and PB is peroneal bre-vis. PM is peroneal muscle. LM is lateral malleoli

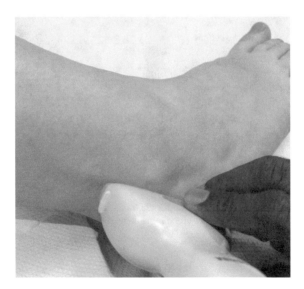

Fig. 30 Patient position and probe position of the longitudinal evaluation of the peroneal tendons

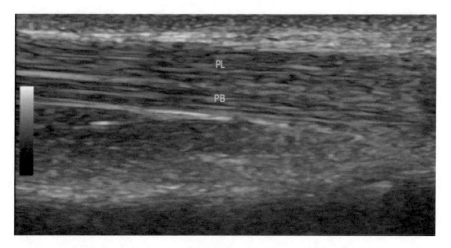

Fig. 31 Longitudinal view of the peroneal tendons. PL is peroneal longus and PB is peroneal brevis. PM is peroneal muscle. LM is lateral malleoli

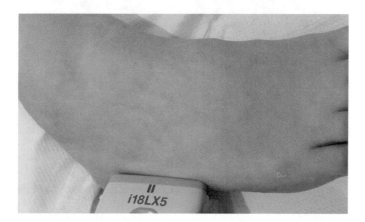

Fig. 32 Patient position and probe position of the longitudinal evaluation of the peroneal tendons insertion of the 5th MT head

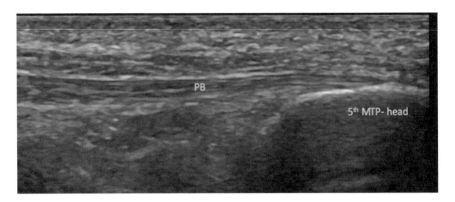

Fig. 33 Longitudinal view of PB insertion on the 5th MT head

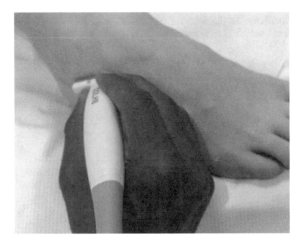

Fig. 34 Patient position and probe position for examination of the anterior talo-fibular joint

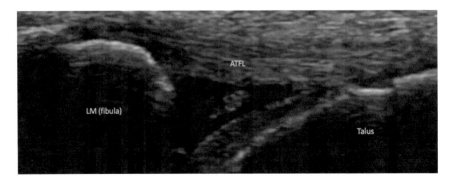

Fig. 35 Longitudinal view of the anterior talo-fibular joint (ATFL)

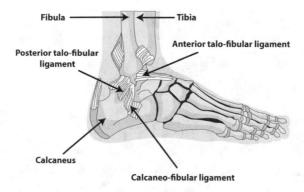

Fibula ——————→   ←—————— Tibia

Anterior talo-fibular ligament

Posterior talo-fibular
ligament

Calcaneus

Calcaneo-fibular ligament

Illustration 9   Diagram of the anterior talo-fibular ligament (ATFL). Figure commissioned by Dr Akram and printed with permission from Unzag Designs

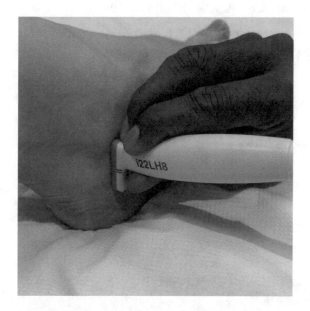

Fig. 36   Patient position and probe position for examination of the calcaneo fibular joint

The, **calcaneo-fibular joint (CTFL) (illustrations 6 and 9)** is then seen in the same position (Figs. 36, 37) with a dorsiflexion of the foot. The probe is then placed on the lateral malleoli to the upper and lateral surface of the calcaneus. The probe is swept from proximal to distal [4].

Forefoot

Keeping the patient in the same position as for examination of the anterior part of the joint, the probe is swept further distally and parallel to the metatarsal bones to

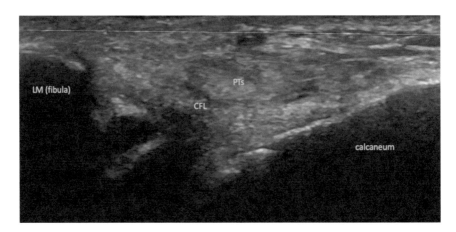

Fig. 37 Longitudinal view of the calcaneo-fibular joint (CTFL)

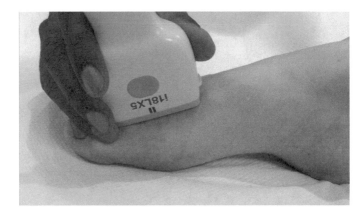

Fig. 38 Patient position and probe position (starting point) for the evaluation of the MTP joints

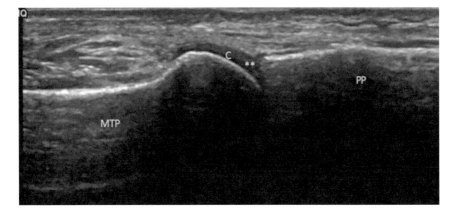

Fig. 39 Longitudinal scan of the MTP joints. MTP is metatarso-phalangeal. PP is proximal phalanx. C is cartilage. ** is the synovium

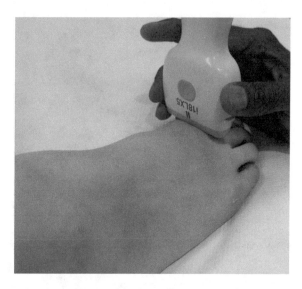

Fig. 40 Patient position and probe position for evaluation of the transverse MTPJ

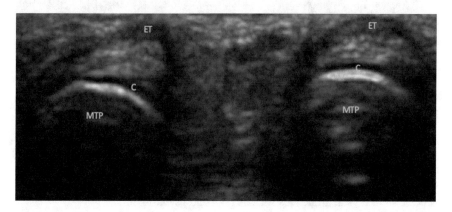

Fig. 41 Transverse evaluation of the MTPJ. MTP is metatarso-phalangeal joint. PP is proximal phalanx. C is cartilage. ** is the synovium. ET is extensor tendon

evaluate the meta-tarsal phalangeal joints (MTPJ) followed by the inter-phalangeal (IP) joints.

The probe is placed in the longitudinal view (Figs. 38, 39) and then in transverse view (Figs. 40, 41). Each MTPJs, proximal interphalangeal joint (PIPJ) and distal interphalangeal joint (DIPJ) is assessed (Figs. 42, 43). Careful examination is made of the bone, cartilage, synovium and overlying extensor tendon [4, 5].

The medial aspect of bone cortex of the 1st MTPJ (Figs. 44, 45) and lateral aspect of 5th MTPJ (Figs. 46, 47) is also assessed in the same position. These are common sites for erosions in rheumatoid arthritis.

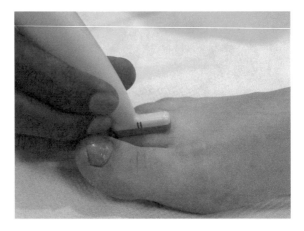

Fig. 42 Patient position and probe position for evaluation of the PIP and DIP joints

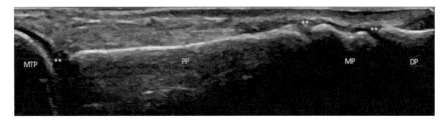

Fig. 43 Longitudinal evaluation of the PIP joints and DIP joints. MTP is metatarso-phalangeal. PP is proximal phalanx. DP is distal phalanx. ** represents the MTPJ and then the IPJ

A transverse view of the MTP cartilage should also made with knee flexed, heel on table, and toes passively flexed. The probe should be swept from medial to lateral. This can be important to identify loss of cartilage in osteoarthritis and crystal deposition in crystal arthritides such as gout and pseudo-gout.

Posterior Ankle

The Achilles tendon is a large tendon that aids the ankle in plantar flexion through the actions of the soleus, plantaris and gastrocnemius muscles on the calcaneum [2, 3].

The examination of the posterior joint (**Illustration 10**) is performed by placing the patient prone, knees fully extended and the leg resting on the examination table. The foot can be placed in a slight dorsiflexion to contract the achilles tendon.

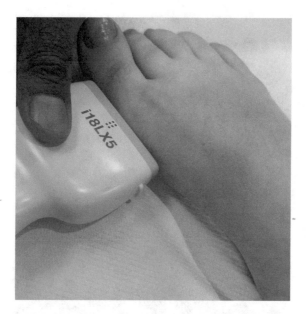

Fig. 44 Patient position and probe position for the evaluation of the lateral 1st MTP joint

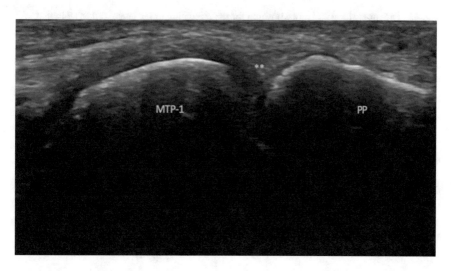

Fig. 45 Longitudinal evaluation of the lateral 1st MTP joint. MTP is metatarso-phalangeal. PP is proximal phalanx. ** is the MTPJ

The transducer is placed in long axis on the **achilles tendon** sweeping the probe proximally (Figs. 48, 49) starting at the muscle–tendon junction and then distally to evaluate the tendon, retrocalcaneal bursa and posterior tibio-talar joint

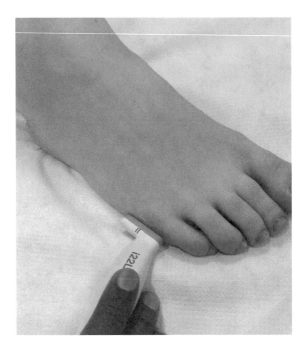

Fig. 46 Patient position and probe position for the evaluation of the lateral 5th MTP joint

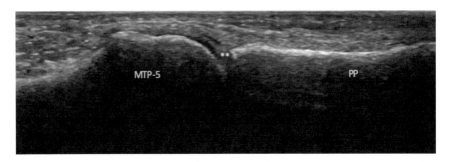

Fig. 47 Longitudinal evaluation of the lateral 1st MTP joint. MTP is metatarso-phalangeal. PP is proximal phalanx. ** is the MTPJ

(Figs. 50, 51). The achilles enthesis (Figs. 52, 53) is then examined carefully and is an important site for diseases such as the spondyloarthopathies. The probe can be rotated 180 degrees to obtain transverse views of the achilles tendon at the enthesis and also at the muscle–tendon junction (Figs. 54, 55, 56, 57) [4].

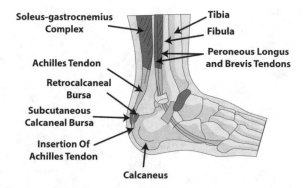

Illustration 10 Illustration of the posterior ankle including the achilles tendon. Figure commissioned by Dr Akram and printed with permission from Unzag Designs

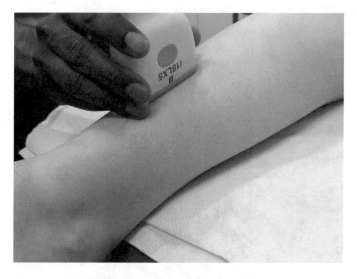

Fig. 48 Patient position and probe position for examination of the longitudinal achilles tendon

Plantar Ankle and Foot

To examine the plantar fascia (Illustration 11) the patient is kept prone and a long axis view of the medial tubercle of calcaneus. For the long axis scan more pressure must be applied on distal edge of the probe. Probe is swept from proximal to distal to get a full view of the plantar fascia (Figs. 58, 59) [4, 5].

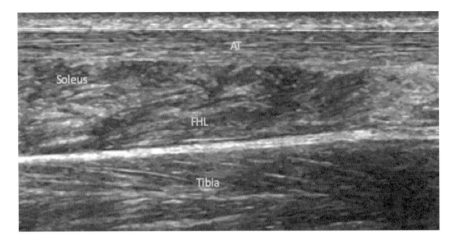

Fig. 49 Longitudinal view of the achilles tendon. Note: soleus and FHL

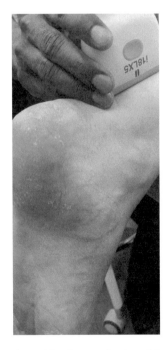

Fig. 50 Patient position and probe position for examination of the longitudinal achilles tendon

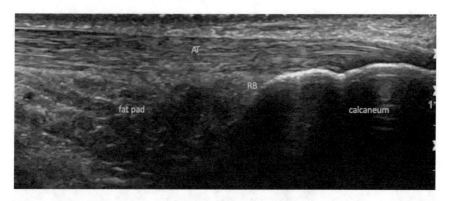

Fig. 51 Longitudinal view of the achilles tendon. Note: retrocalcaneal bursa and posterior recess and tibio-talar joint

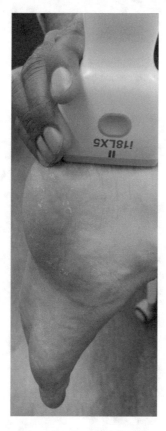

Fig. 52 Patient position and probe position for examination of the longitudinal achilles tendon insertion on the calcaneum

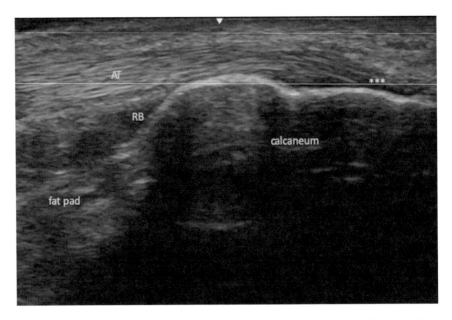

Fig. 53 Longitudinal view of the achilles tendon including insertion on the calcaneum. Note: retrocalcaneal bursa and posterior recess and tibio-talar joint. **** is the insertion of the achilles tendon

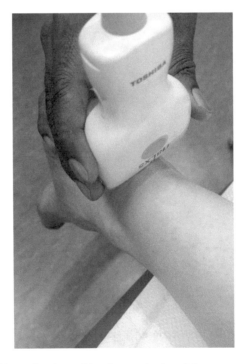

Fig. 54 Patient position and probe position for examination of the transverse achilles tendon

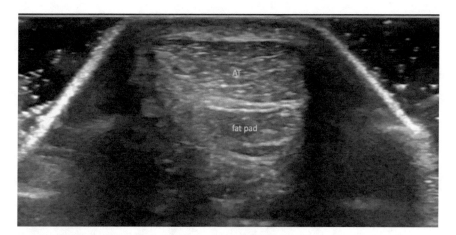

Fig. 55 Transverse view of the achilles tendon including the Kager's fat pad inferior to the tendon

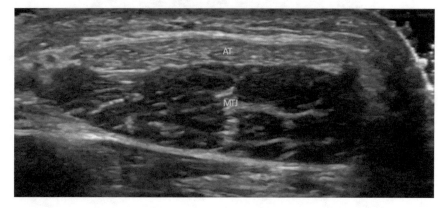

Fig. 56 Patient position and probe position for examination of the transverse achilles tendon at the level of the myotendinous junction

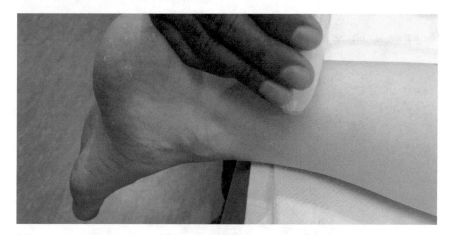

Fig. 57 Transverse view of the achilles tendon at the level of the myotendinous junction

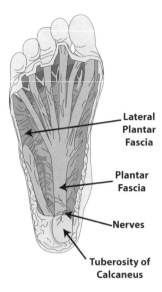

Illustration 11   Illustration of the plantar fascia. Figure commissioned by Dr Akram and printed with permission from Unzag Designs

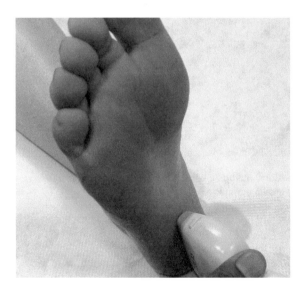

Fig. 58   Patient position and probe position for examination of the plantar fascia

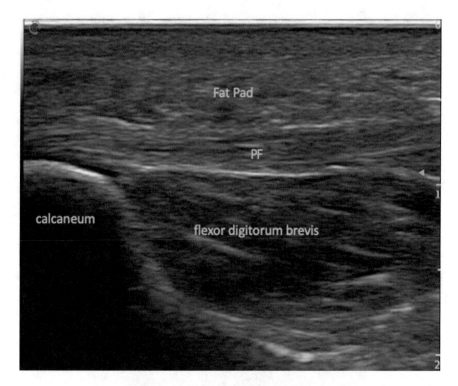

Fig. 59 Longitudinal view of the plantar fascia. PF is the plantar fascia

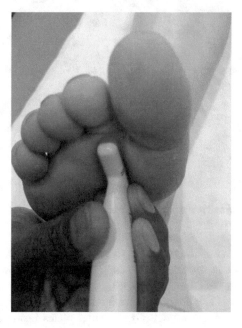

Fig. 60 Patient position and probe position for examination of the longitudinal flexor digitorum longus tendon

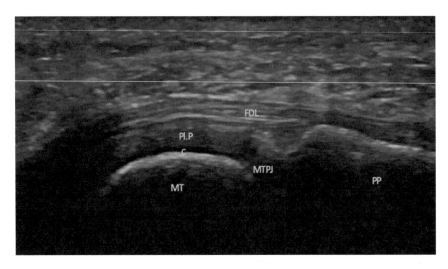

Fig. 61 Longitudinal view of the flexor digitorum longus tendon. MT is metatarsal. FDL is flexor digitorum longus. PlP is plantar plate. C is cartilage

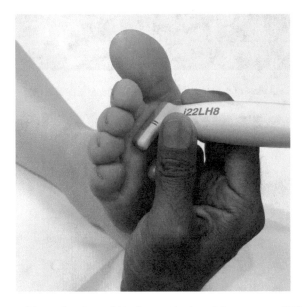

Fig. 62 Patient position and probe position for examination of the transverse MTPJ

The **flexor digitorum longus (FDL) tendon** is then examined by asking the patient to place foot in dorsiflexion. A long axis scan is done on plantar aspect of foot parallel to the MT bones (Figs. 60, 61). Then a transverse scan (Figs. 62, 63) should performed. The flexor digitorum longus and the flexor digitorum brevis tendons run on the inferior aspect of the plantar plates inside a common fibrous

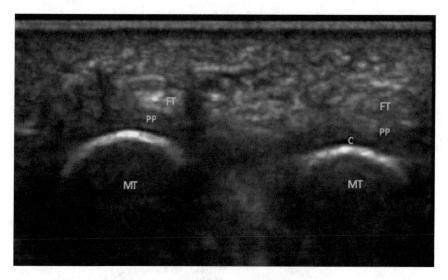

Fig. 63 Transverse examination of the MTPJ. MP is metatarsal phalanx. C is cartilage. PP is plantar plate. FT is flexor tendon

sheath invested by a synovial membrane. The sheath is composed of anterior insertion of the plantar facia and by its transverse fibres (Illustration 11) [4].

The interdigital spaces, common sites for neuromas and bursitis, can also be viewed at this position as shown with the probe in transverse and being swept from medial to lateral (Figs. 64, 65).

Pathology

The reason for using ultrasound in rheumatology is to detect abnormal pathology which can enable an accurate diagnosis especially at the point of care. The foot and ankle are the most frequent sites to be involved in rheumatological disease.

The evaluation of the tibio-talar, subtalar, anterior and lateral recesses, mid tarsal joints and the MTPJ, PIPJs and DIPJs can detect effusion or synovitis/synovial hypertrophy. This may also have a positive power doppler signal. This is usually present in inflammatory arthritis such as rheumatoid arthritis, spondyloarthropathy, crystal arthritis, inflammatory osteoarthritis and septic arthritis (Figs. 66, 67, 68, 69, 70, 71, 72, 73) [6, 7].

An assessment of the tendons at both ankle and foot level (including the extensor tendon compartments and flexor tendons) and ligaments can detect tenosynovitis, enthesopathy or tears. This is usually caused by spondyloarthropathy or rheumatoid arthritis. Mechanical overuse or trauma may cause tendon or ligament tears. Tendon and ligament tears may be observed as an anechoic or hypoechoic

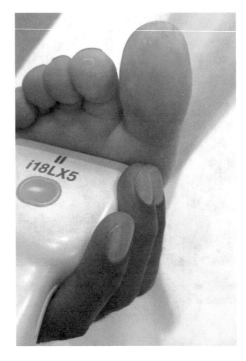

Fig. 64 Patient position and probe position for examination of the interdigital spaces

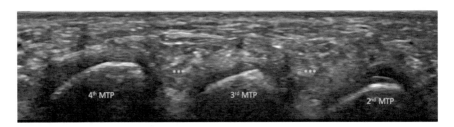

Fig. 65 Transverse view of the interdigital spaces. MTP is the metatarsophalanx. *** is the interdigital space

discontinuity of the fibrillary pattern with or without retraction and, in recent cases, with surrounding hypoechoic fluid (Figs. 74, 75, 76, 77, 78) [6].

An examination of the joints especially the mid tarsal and MTPJs can identify erosions can be seen (Figs. 79, 80). The PIPJs and DIPs can also be affected.

Osteoarthritis causes characteristic osteophytes which can be seen at the DIPJ, PIPJs and MTPJs (Figs. 80, 81, 82, 83). The hyaline cartilage can be thinned. Spondyloarthopathies (Fig. 84) such as psoriatic arthritis can affect the DIPJs

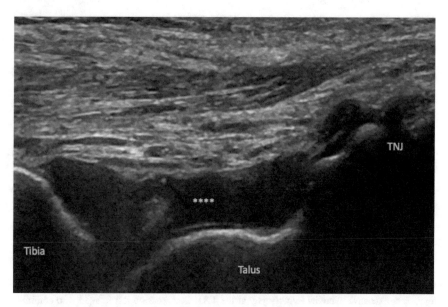

Fig. 66 Longitudinal view of the tibio-talar joint in a patient with rheumatoid arthritis. ****
represents extensive synovial hypertrophy. Compression test is needed to confirm if this shows
presence of an effusion. TNJ is talo-navicular joint

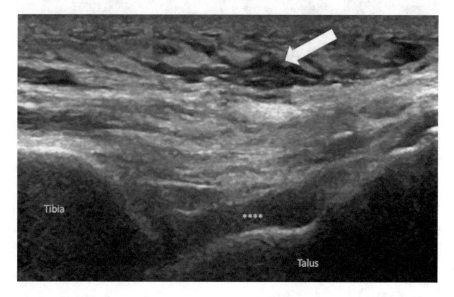

Fig. 67 Longitudinal view of the tibio-talar joint in a patient with rheumatoid arthritis. ****
represents extensive synovial hypertrophy. Compression test is needed to confirm if this shows
presence of an effusion. TNJ is talo-navicular joint. White arrow shoes extensive subcutaneous
oedema

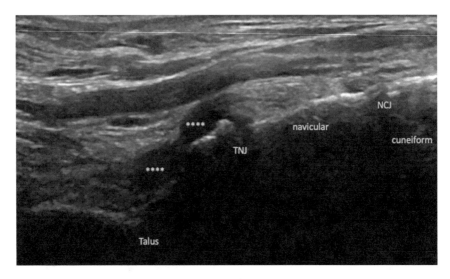

Fig. 68 Longitudinal view of the mid tarsal joint in a patient with rheumatoid arthritis. ****
represents extensive synovial hypertrophy at the TNJ. Compression test is needed to confirm if
this shows presence of an effusion. TNJ is talo-navicular joint. NCJ is naviculo-cuneiform joint

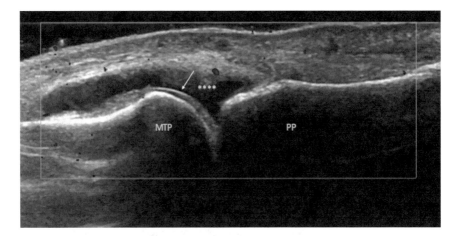

Fig. 69 Longitudinal view of the 1st MTP joint in a patient with rheumatoid arthritis. *** represents extensive synovial hypertrophy at the TNJ. Compression test is needed to confirm if this
shows presence of an effusion. White arrow shows fluid interface sign and not to be confused
with the double contour sign seen in gout

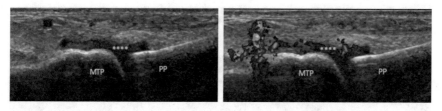

Fig. 70 Longitudinal view of the 1st MTP joint in a patient with rheumatoid arthritis. **a** shows in grey scale and **b** in power doppler mode. **** represents extensive synovial hypertrophy

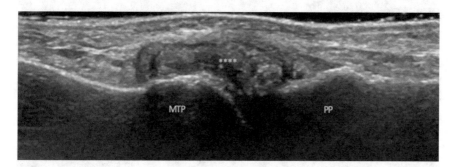

Fig. 71 Longitudinal view of the 1st MTP joint in a patient with rheumatoid arthritis. *** represents extensive synovial hypertrophy

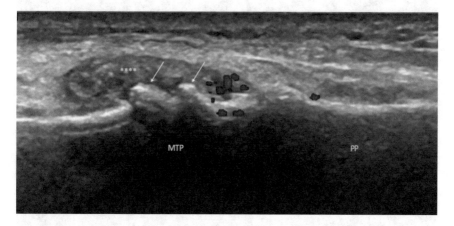

Fig. 72 Longitudinal view of the 1st MTP joint in a patient with rheumatoid arthritis. **** represents synovial hypertrophy. White arrows indicate osteophytes. There is a combination of inflammatory arthritis and osteoarthritis

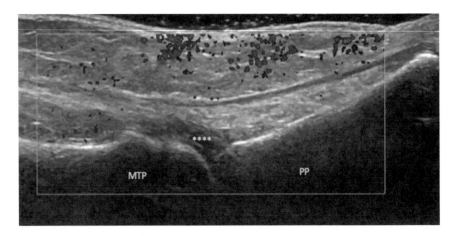

Fig. 73 Longitudinal view of the 2nd MTP joint in a patient with rheumatoid arthritis. *** represents extensive synovial hypertrophy

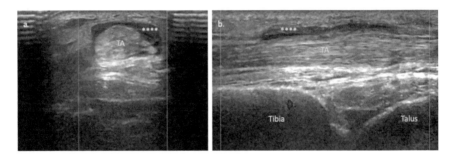

Fig. 74 Transverse (**a**) and Longitudinal (**b**). views of the Tibialis Anterior tendon demonstrating tenosynovitis in a patient with rheumatoid arthritis. **** represents tenosynovitis

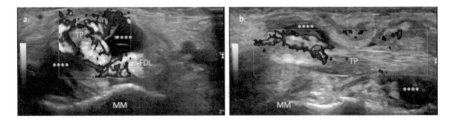

Fig. 75 Transverse (**a**) and Longitudinal (**b**) views of the Tibialis posterior tendon demonstrating tenosynovitis (with doppler activity) in a patient with rheumatoid arthritis. **** represents tenosynovitis. MM is medial malleolus. TP is tibialis posterior tendon. FDL is flexor digitorum longus

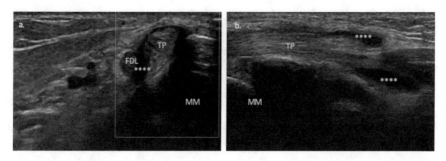

Fig. 76 Transverse (**a**) and Longitudinal (**b**) views of the Tibialis posterior tendon demonstrating tenosynovitis (with doppler activity) in a patient with rheumatoid arthritis. **** represents tenosynovitis. MM is medial malleolus. TP is tibialis posterior tendon. FDL is flexor digitorum longus

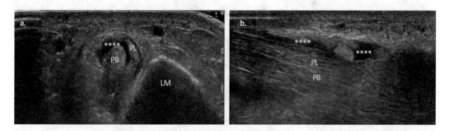

Fig. 77 Transverse (**a**) and Longitudinal (**b**) views of the peroneal tendons demonstrating tenosynovitis in a patient with rheumatoid arthritis. **** represents tenosynovitis. LM is lateral malleolus. PB is peroneal brevis and PL is peroneal longus

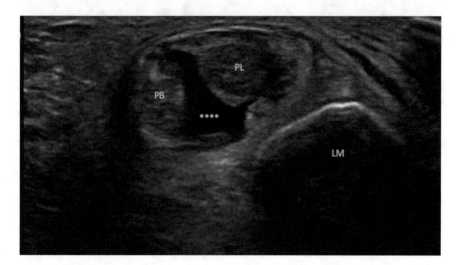

Fig. 78 Transverse views of the peroneal tendons demonstrating tenosynovitis in a patient with rheumatoid arthritis. **** represents tenosynovitis. LM is lateral malleolus. PB is peroneal brevis and PL is peroneal longus

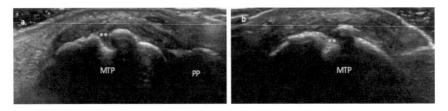

Fig. 79 **a** Longitudinal and **b** Transverse view of the 1st MTPJ in a patient with rheumatoid arthritis. MTP is metatarso-phalanx. PP is proximal phalanx. ** is erosion of the MTP

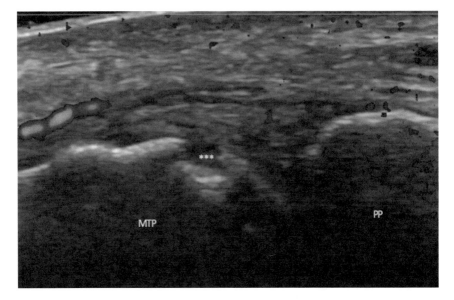

Fig. 80 Longitudinal view of the 1st MTPJ in a patient with rheumatoid arthritis. MTP is meta-tarso-phalanx. PP is proximal phalanx. ** is erosion of the MTP

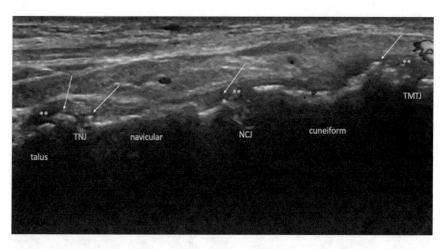

Fig. 81 Longitudinal view of the mid tarsal joint in a patient with osteoarthritis. ** represents synovial hypertrophy associated with osteophytes (white arrows). TNJ is talo-navicular joint. NCJ is naviculo-cuneiform joint. TMTJ is tarso-metatarsal joint

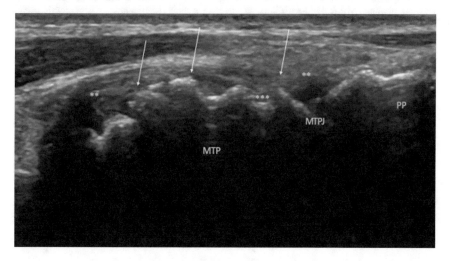

Fig. 82 Longitudinal view of the 1st MTPJ in a patient with osteoarthritis. MTP is metatarso-phalanx. PP is proximal phalanx. White arrows show osteophytes. ** is synovitis associated with osteophyte. *** shows a possible erosion due to osteoarthritis

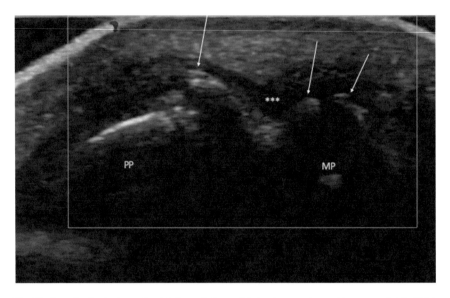

Fig. 83 Longitudinal view of a 4th interphalangeal joint in a patient with osteoarthritis. PP is proximal phalanx. MP is middle phalanx. White arrows show osteophytes. ** is synovitis associated with osteophyte

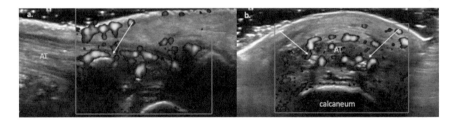

Fig. 84 **a** Longitudinal and **a** Transverse view of the achilles tendon in a patient with Spondyloarthropathy. White arrows show calcifications in the tendon. Power doppler activity suggesting active disease. AT is achilles tendon

whereas rheumatoid arthritis will only affect as far up to the PIPJs. Although, beyond the scope of this book nail involvement can also be seen in psoriatic arthritis on ultrasound [6].

Crystal arthritis commonly affects the foot and ankles (crystals precipitate in cooler areas) including both monosodium urate gout and calcium pyrophosphate disease. These can commonly be seen at sites as a bright hyperechoic area and the

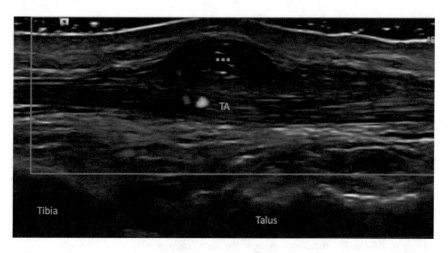

Fig. 85 Longitudinal view of the tibialis anterior showing gouty tophus *** in. a patient with gout

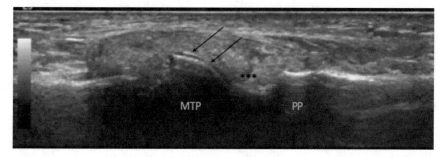

Fig. 86 Longitudinal view of the 1st MTPJ in a patient with gout. MTP is metatarso-phalanx. PP is proximal phalanx. Black arrows show double contour sign

hyaline cartilage of the MTPJs especially the 1st MTPJ as a double contour sign. Tophi can also be seen at the level of the interphalangeal joints (Figs. 85, 86, 87). Pseudogout can be deposited within the hyaline cartilage and seen as a rose beading sign [6].

An assessment of the tibial nerve can demonstrate common pathologies such as tarsal tunnel syndrome, similar to carpal tunnel syndrome, commonly caused by ankle synovitis.

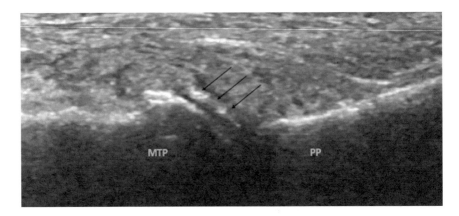

Fig. 87 Longitudinal view of the 1st MTPJ in a patient with gout. MTP is metatarso-phalanx. PP is proximal phalanx. Black arrows show double contour sign

References

1. Hansen JT. Lower limb. Netter's clinical anatomy, Chapter 7, pp. 367–435. Elsevier; 2018.
2. Paulsen F. Lower extremity. In: Sobotta Atlas of Human Anatomy, Vol.1, 3, 127–242. Urban and Fischer; 2013.
3. Drake RL, Waze Vogla A, Mitchell AVM. Gray's basic anatomy, 2nd ed. Elsevier; 2017.
4. Bianchi S, Martinoli C. Ultrasound of the musculo-skeletal system. Springer; 2007.
5. Filippucci E, Iagnocco A, Meenagh G, et al. Ultrasound imaging for the rheumatologist II. Ultrasonography of the foot and ankle. Clin Exp Rheumatol. 2006;24:118–22.
6. Wakefield RJ, Balint PV, Szkudlarek M et al. OMERACT 7 special interest group. Musculoskeletal ultrasound including definitions for ultrasonographic pathology. J Rheumatol. 2005;32(12):2485–7.
7. Moller I, Janta I, Backhaus M, et al. The 2017 EULAR standardized procedures for ultrasound imaging in rheumatology. Ann Rheum Dis. 2017;76(12):1974–9.

Ultrasound in Large Vessel Vasculitis

Anne Christine Bull Haaversen and Andreas P. Diamantopoulos

Basics of Vascular Ultrasound

The Outcome Measures in Rheumatology (OMERACT) group on ultrasound in large vessel vasculitides (LVV) has developed definitions and standardized the ultrasonographic findings of inflammation in temporal and axillary arteritis [3]. Cut-offs for the normal thickness in cranial and axillary arteries have been developed, mainly to distinguish vasculitis from atherosclerosis (Table 1) [4].

We suggest the examination of the temporal artery in two planes when the halo sign appears to be present. Compression sign should always apply in short axis to avoid false negatives (the inflamed artery can slide to the side if compressed in the long axis). For the large vessels, examination in long axis is sufficient.

The Fast Track ultrasound GCA clinics reduce significantly the number of patients suffering from irreversible visual loss [5, 6] and have been introduced in many countries thus improving outcomes for GCA patients.

The anteromedial ultrasound examination technique which is demonstrated in this chapter includes a complete and systematic examination of the supra-aortic tree, the aortic arch, the ascending and the abdominal aorta in all LVV patients (Table 2). Preliminary results have demonstrated the superiority of the anteromedial ultrasound examination in the identification of large-vessel involvement in GCA patients (up to 79% of all GCA patients) [7]. Additionally, we use the anteromedial ultrasound approach as a diagnostic and follow-up tool for all GCA and TAK patients. Furthermore, ultrasound is used to confirm a flare or to evaluate response to treatment (Table 2). The anteromedial approach requires a recording

A. C. B. Haaversen (✉) · A. P. Diamantopoulos
Department of Rheumatology, Martina Hansens Hospital, Bærum, Dønskiveien 8, 1346 Gjettum, Norway
e-mail: annecbull@gmail.com

A. P. Diamantopoulos
e-mail: adiamanteas@gmail.com

© The Author(s), under exclusive license to Springer Nature Switzerland AG 2021
Q. Akram and S. Basu (eds.), *Ultrasound in Rheumatology*,
https://doi.org/10.1007/978-3-030-68659-8_8

Table 1 Overview of the cut-off values for the cranial and axillary arteries [4, 19]

Artery	Cut-off values (mm)
Temporal artery common superficial	0.42
Temporal artery frontal branch	0.34
Temporal artery parietal branch	0.29
Facial artery	0.37
Axillary artery	1.00

Table 2 Flowchart of the suggested ultrasound evaluation of LVV patients

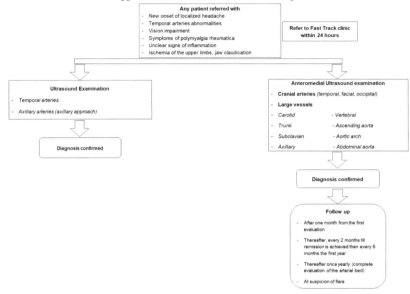

of the vasculitic changes and a comparison between consequent examinations to identify differences in IMT (for the response to treatment, damage or disease flare) [8].

Definitions

Intima media thickness (IMT) is the "area of tissue starting at the luminal edge of the artery and ending at the boundary between the media and the adventitia" [9]. Any transducer >15 MHz for the cranial arteries and >10 MHz for the supra-aortic arteries should be sufficient for the proper visualization of the arteries [1, 10]. To examine the aorta, a phased array transducer for the ascending aorta and the aortic arch and a curvilinear transducer for the abdominal aorta and the deep pelvic vessels are considered sufficient [1, 10].

OMERACT Ultrasound Working Group in large vessel vasculitis standardized the definitions of vasculitic vessel wall changes (halo sign) and compression sign and tested the reliability of the developed definitions [3, 11]. OMERACT has defined the 'halo sign' as "a homogeneous, hypoechoic wall thickening well-delineated towards the luminal side visible both in longitudinal and transverse planes, most commonly concentric in transverse planes" [3]. The compression sign helps to distinguish inflammation of the vessel wall in cranial arteries from pseudo halo due to incorrect ultrasound equipment adjustments or poor technique [12]. According to the OMERACT definition, "The thickened arterial wall remains visible upon compression, i.e. the echogenicity contrasts hypoechoic due to vasculitis vessel wall thickening in comparison to the mid-to hyperechoic surrounding tissue" [3] (Fig. 21c).

The use of cut-off values for IMT of the cranial and axillary arteries may be useful to distinguish vasculitis from normal arteries in patients suspected to have GCA [4]. The cut-off values are presented in Table 1.

Atherosclerosis which is one of the main challenges in ultrasound in vasculitis is defined as hypo-, iso- or hyperechoic, non-homogeneous and localized plaques seen mainly in the large vessels at bifurcations. In some patients, atherosclerosis may present as an iso- or hyperechoic, homogeneous wall thickening thus making difficult the distinction from chronic vasculitic changes (Fig. 23). In rare cases in the cranial vessels, a biopsy may be necessary to distinguish vasculitis from atherosclerosis.

It is important to note that halo sign is not a distinct feature of GCA, but can appear in other vasculitides (ANCA associated vasculitides, polyarteritis nodosa), infections, or other rare conditions [13–15].

Ultrasonographically, there are no differences in echogenicity in TAK patients compared to GCA patients. The slope sign is a pathologically increased IMT that spreads over a long arterial segment and slides down to a normal brachial artery and is mainly observed in GCA patients [16, 17] (Fig. 29b).

Observational cohort studies demonstrated the distinct differences regarding the distribution of vasculitic involvement among GCA and TAK. GCA involves predominantly the cranial, subclavian and axillary arteries, while TAK involves the left carotid, the left subclavian and the abdominal arteries [18].

Settings and Pitfalls

Gray Scale

Now, moving to the ultrasound examination of the arterial system, the depth of the image should be kept at 1–1.5 cm for the temporal artery and at 2–2.5 for the facial and occipital arteries. For the supraaortic arteries, the depth should be sufficient to visualize the artery in the middle of the screen. Brightness should be enough to visualize the vessel wall and can be adjusted by the B mode gain. An image that is too bright, may lead to the incorrect conclusion that the increased IMT is atherosclerotic while too dark, images may miss the inflammatory changes of the vessel wall. Frequency should be adjusted according to the depth in which the vessel is localized. Superficial vessels require higher frequencies, while deeper vessels lower frequencies.

Color Doppler

Color Doppler has the advantage of visualizing the blood flow direction thus improving the diagnostic capability of ultrasound especially if stenosis and occlusion are present. Color Doppler is preferred for the visualization of the cranial arteries and if stenosis or occlusion are suspected in the large vessels. In Color Doppler the angle of insonation of the Doppler window should be preferably kept between 30 and 60 degrees and in any case < 90 degrees to avoid inadequate filling of the arterial lumen. In addition, the color Doppler gain should be adjusted so the color fills the lumen completely (Fig. 1).

Pulse Repetition Frequency (PRF) is one of the important adjustments in vascular ultrasound. PRF is the number of ultrasound pulses emitted by the transducer over a designated period of time. For the examination of the cranial arteries, a PRF of 2–3 MHz is sufficient while for the large vessels a higher value of 4 MHz is adequate.

Pitfalls

Blooming Appears when the color exceeds beyond the artery walls. The reason for blooming is that the color gain is too high or PRF is too low (Fig. 21).
Solution: Adjust the color gain and PRF accordingly.

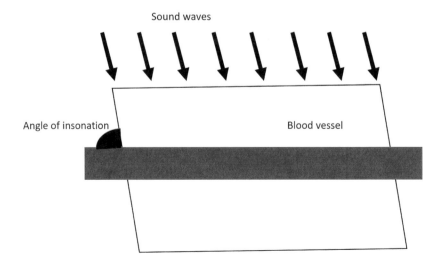

Fig. 1 Angle of insonation

Pseudo halo. In pseudo halo, the thickened area appears anechoic and this should alert the ultrasonographer of the possibility of wrong adjustments as vasculitis appears hypoechoic and fluid (in this case the blood flow) anechoic (Fig. 22). Pseudo halo appears if the color gain is low, the PRF is very high or if the Color Box is not steered properly. Pseudo halo is also observed in areas of hair such as the scalp especially in the parietal area.

Solution: Raise the gain, reduce the PRF to approximately 2. 5 kHz or steer the color box appropriately in order for the sound waves to meet the blood flow at an angle between 30 and 60 degrees (Fig. 1). In hairy areas use copious amounts of gel. However, the most practical solution to avoid pseudo halo is to compress the artery. In the case of a positive compression sign, the residual hypoechoic tissue after the compression is the thickened inflamed arterial wall (Fig. 24c).

Ultrasonographic Atlas of Examination of the Cranial Arteries, the Supraaortic Arteries and the Aorta

A. Cranial Arteries

See Fig. 2.

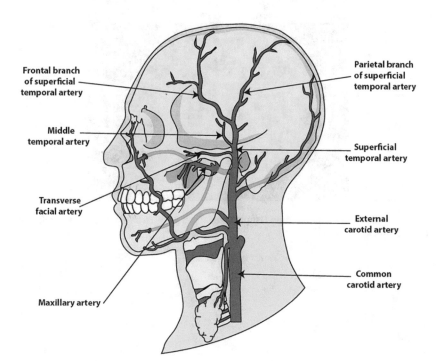

Fig. 2 Anatomical overview of the cranial vessels

Temporal Artery

The examination of the temporal arteries begins with the transducer longitudinally in front of the ear (Fig. 3a,b). It continues towards the parietal branch (Fig. 4a,b) until the top of the head and then turns transversely to the bifurcation. The frontal artery should be identified longitudinally and followed up to the frontal area (Fig. 5a,b) and then transversely backward to the bifurcation. The examination ends with a transverse view of the common branch.

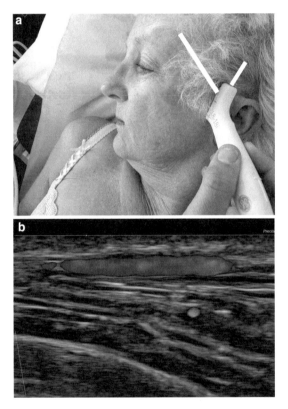

Fig. 3 Examination of the **common temporal artery**: **a** position of the transducer, **b** ultrasound image, longitudinal view

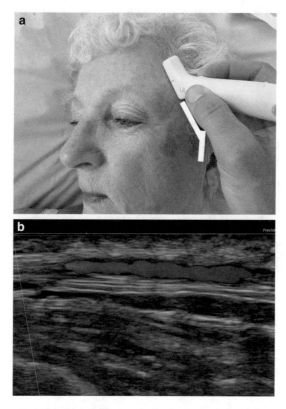

Fig. 4 Examination of the **frontal temporal artery**: **a** recommended position of the transducer **b** ultrasound image, longitudinal view

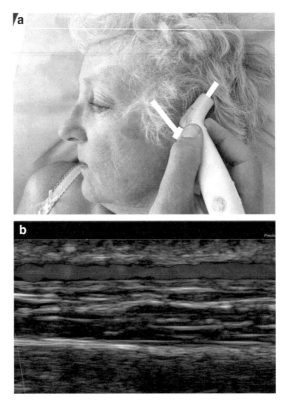

Fig. 5 Examination of the **parietal branch** of the temporal artery: **a** recommended position of the transducer, **b** ultrasound image, longitudinal view

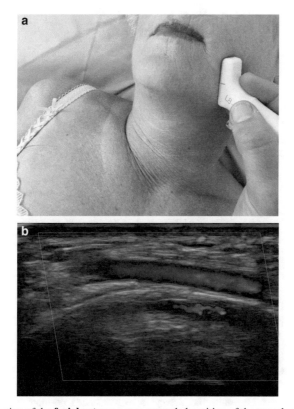

Fig. 6 Examination of the **facial artery**: **a** recommended position of the transducer **b** ultrasound image, longitudinal view

Distal Facial Artery

The examination starts with the identification of the facial artery in a transverse view in the middle of the jaw and continuing proximally towards the ear (Fig. 6).

Occipital Artery

The occipital artery is identified just below the mastoid process (Fig. 7) and should be followed longitudinally towards the back of the head.

B. **Ultrasonographic Examination of the Supraaortic Arteries**

The examination of the supraaortic arteries requires the use of medium frequency probes to visualize the deep vessels (e.g. subclavian, vertebral). The phased array probe should be used to examine the ascending aorta, the aortic arch, and the

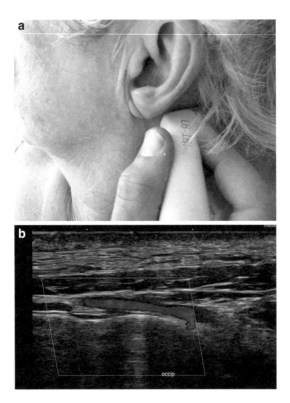

Fig. 7 Examination of the **occipital artery**: **a** recommended position of the transducer **b** ultrasound image, longitudinal view

aortic valve. The low-frequency curvilinear probe is an excellent choice for the visualization of the abdominal aorta and the deep pelvic arteries.

The examination starts by visualizing the carotid artery in the short axis in the middle of the neck. An important point here is the identification of the internal and external carotid artery and the use of Doppler to assure that blood flow is present.

Anatomically, the axillary artery is divided into 3 parts according to its relation to the pectoralis minor muscle (first part proximal or suprapectoral, second part behind or subscapular and the third part or infrapectoral distal to pectoralis minor).

However, for practical reasons, we divide ultrasonographically the axillary artery into two segments with the subscapular artery being the turning point: one proximal (from clavicle to the subscapular artery) and one distal (from subscapular to the deep brachial artery) (Figs. 8 and 9).

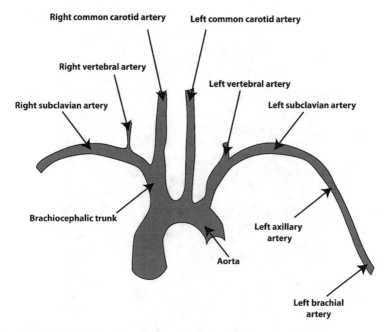

Fig. 8 Anatomical overview of the supraaortic arteries and aorta

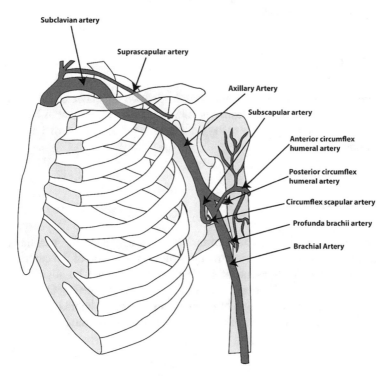

Fig. 9 Anatomical overview of supraaortic arteries, left side

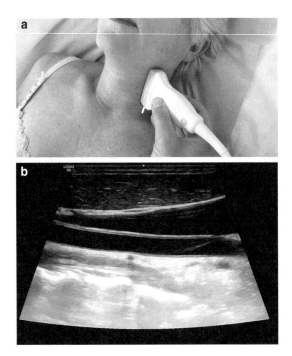

Fig. 10 Examination of the **carotid artery**: **a** recommended transducer position, **b** ultrasonographic image, longitudinal view

Carotid Artery

The examination in the middle of the neck just above the clavicle with the transducer placed transversely. The artery is followed in its whole length both proximally to the clavicle and distally to the skull base. Internal and external arteries are also identified (Fig. 10).

Vertebral Artery

The vertebral artery is localized posteriorly and lateral to the carotid artery. Visualization of the vertebral artery requires the identification of the carotid artery in a longitudinal view. Subsequently, the transducer should be slightly pointed laterally until the vertebral artery is identified (Fig. 11). Color Doppler should be used to identify the artery. The color in the vertebral artery should be compared to the color of the carotid artery to rule out subclavian steal syndrome.

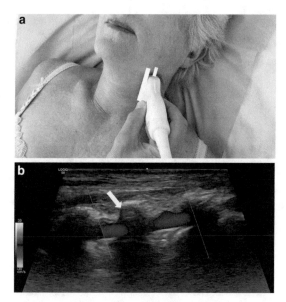

Fig. 11 Examination of the **vertebral artery**: **a** recommended transducer position, **b** ultrasonographic view of the vertebral artery, passing through the vertebra (white arrow)

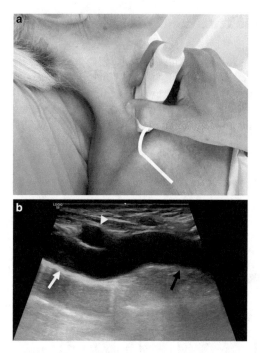

Fig. 12 Examination of the **right subclavian artery**: **a** recommended transducer position, **b** ultrasonographic view of the brachiocephalic trunk (black arrow), carotid artery (arrowhead), subclavian artery (white arrow)

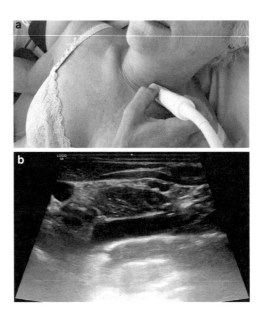

Fig. 13 Examination of the **left subclavian artery**: **a** recommended transducer position, **b** ultrasonographic view of the left subclavian artery

Brachiocephalic Trunk and Subclavian Artery

The carotid artery is followed with the transducer proximally in a transverse plane. When the transducer is in contact with the clavicle orientated slightly towards the lung the brachiocephalic trunk arises longitudinally at the right side (Fig. 12) and the subclavian artery at the left side (Fig. 13). The subclavian artery should be followed distally to the proximal edge of the clavicle.

Subclavian Artery

See Fig. 13.

Proximal Axillary Artery

The examination starts with the distal part of the subclavian artery visualized and the transducer in contact with the bony area of the clavicle, the transducer should be moved over the clavicle and placed in the sulcus between the deltoid and the pectoralis muscles (Fig. 14) until the subscapular artery which appears at the lower arterial wall (Fig. 14b).

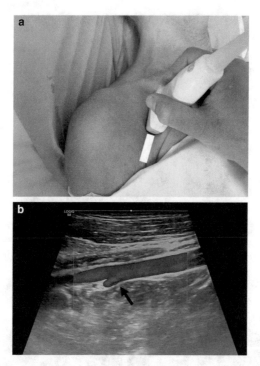

Fig. 14 Examination of the proximal axillary artery: **a** recommended transducer position, **b** ultrasonographic view (subscapular artery-black arrow)

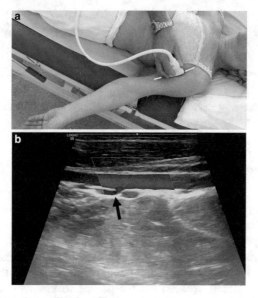

Fig. 15 Examination of the **distal axillary artery**: **a** recommended transducer position, anteromedial approach **b** ultrasonographic view of the distal axillary and brachial artery (including the deep brachial artery-black arrow)

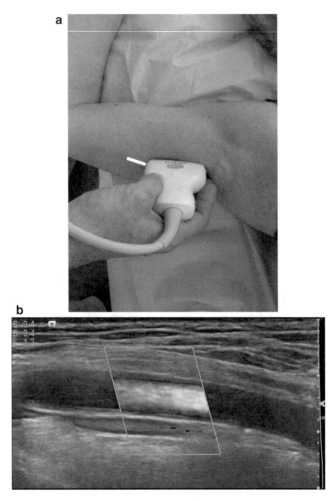

Fig. 16 Examination of the **distal axillary artery,** axillary approach: **a** recommended transducer position, **b** ultrasonographic view of the distal axillary and brachial artery (including the deep brachial artery-black arrow)

Distal Axillary Artery

The distal axillary artery appears after the subscapular artery, by moving the transducer anteromedially (Fig. 15). The artery is visualized through the biceps muscle and appears deeper compared to the axillary scanning. Both the upper and lower vessel wall are pictured. The axillary approach allows the demonstration of the axillary artery with great detail due to the superficial position of the axillary artery. The transducer is placed between the biceps and triceps muscles longitudinally (Fig. 16). However, because of the reverberation artifacts, the upper vessel wall is

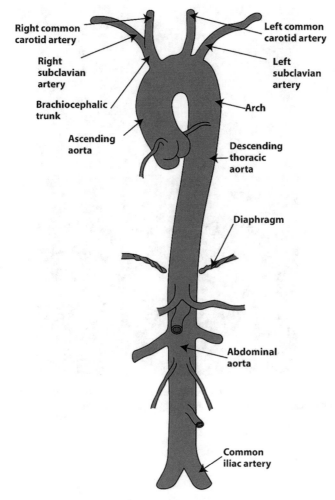

Fig. 17 Overview of the aortic tree

not visible, and the use of color Doppler is strongly advised to identify vasculitic involvement of the upper wall (Fig. 17).

C. **Aorta**

The visualization of the aorta requires the use of lower frequency transducers. The ascending aorta can be visualized by using a phased array transducer in the left parasternal longitudinal view (Fig. 18) and the aortic arch in the suprasternal notch view (Fig. 19). To examine the abdominal aorta the use of a curvilinear low-frequency transducer is advised. The abdominal aorta is identified by using the subcostal approach (Fig. 20) in a transverse view and then switching to a longitudinal view by moving the transducer towards the umbilicus. The bifurcation with both

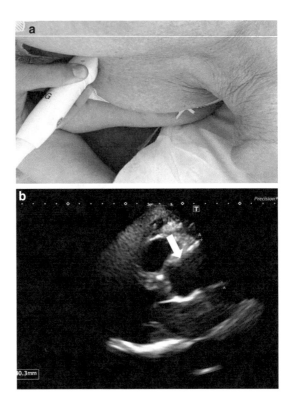

Fig. 18 Examination of the ascending aorta and the aortic valve: **a** recommended transducer position, **b** ultrasonographic view of the ascending aorta (white arrow)

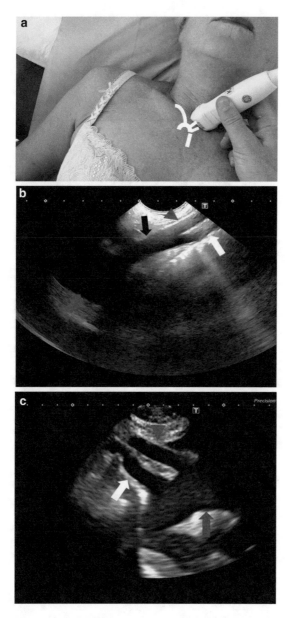

Fig. 19 Examination of the **aortic arch**: **a** recommended transducer position, **b** ultrasonographic view of the brachiocephalic trunk (black arrow), carotid artery (red arrowhead), subclavian artery (white arrow), aorta (red arrow), right side **c** carotid and subclavian artery, aorta, left side

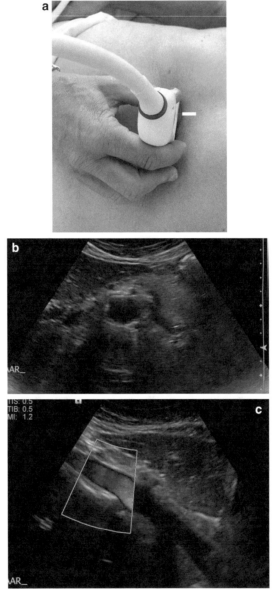

Fig. 20 Examination of **the abdominal aorta**: **a** recommended transducer position, **b** ultrasonographic image, transverse view **c** ultrasonographic image, longitudinal view

the common iliac arteries should be identified. The descending aorta is not satisfactorily visualized by transthoracic ultrasonographic examination.

D. **Pitfalls**

See Fig. 21, 22, and 23.

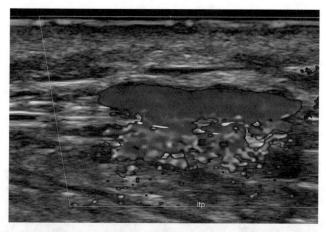

Fig. 21 Blooming: Excessive color which covers the vessel wall

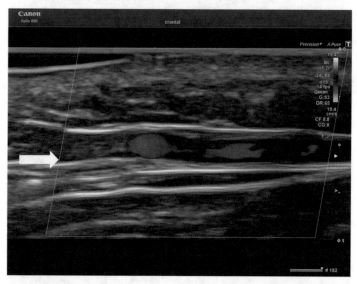

Fig. 22 Pseudohalo. Anechoic halo due to low color Doppler gain, high PRF or wrong angle of insonation (white arrow). The color doesn't fill the vessel lumen completely

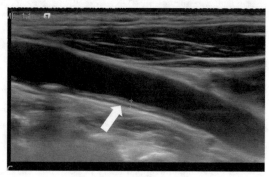

Fig. 23 Atherosclerosis in the carotid artery (white arrow)

Pathology

A. Cranial Arteries

See Figs. 24 and 25.

B. Supraaortic Arteries

See Fig. 26, 27, 28, 29, 30, and 31.

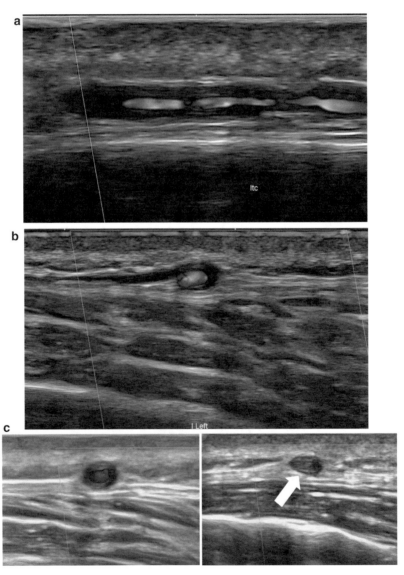

Fig. 24 Increased IMT in the common temporal artery in new-onset GCA. **a** Longitudinal, **b** transverse view **c** positive compression sign (white arrow)

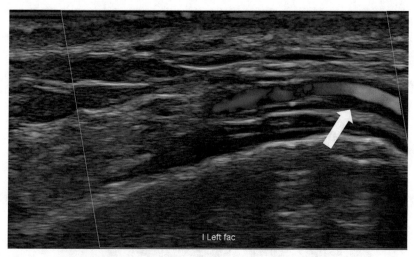

Fig. 25 Increased IMT in the facial artery, longitudinal view (white arrow)

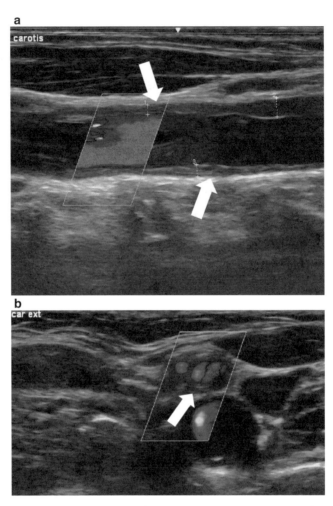

Fig. 26 Increased IMT in new-onset GCA: **a** in the common carotid artery **b** external carotid artery (white arrows)

Fig. 27 Increased IMT in the vertebral artery (white arrow)

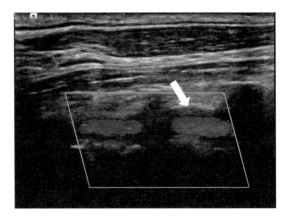

Fig. 28 Increased IMT in **a** the left subclavian artery, **b** the right subclavian artery

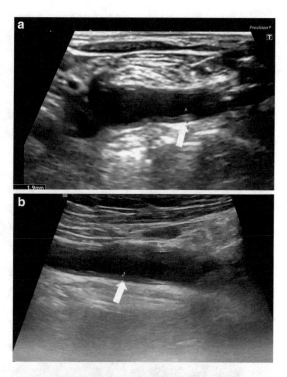

Fig. 29 Axillary arteritis (white arrow) in a GCA patient (axillary imaging approach) **a** distal axillary artery, **b** distal axillary artery, slope sign (white arrowhead at the distal part of the artery)

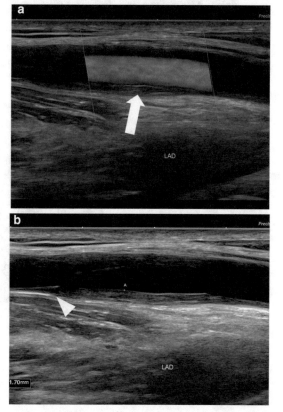

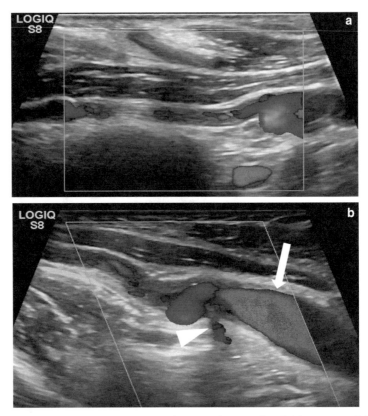

Fig. 30 Axillary artery occlusion in a patient with longstanding GCA (anteromedial imaging approach) **a** distal axillary artery, **b** proximal axillary artery. Note the area of aneurysm in the proximal axillary artery (white arrow) at the subscapular artery area (white arrowhead)

Fig. 31 Increased IMT measured at 5 mm in the aortic arch of a patient with new-onset GCA

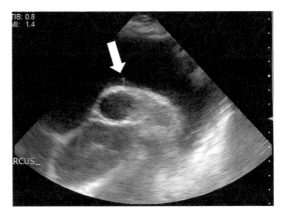

Other Vasculitides

See Fig. 32.

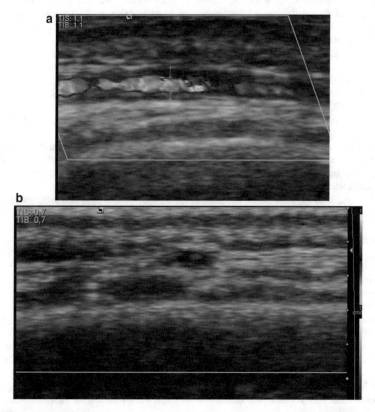

Fig. 32 Increased IMT in the parietal branch of the temporal artery in **a** granulomatosis with polyangiitis **b** polyarteritis nodosa

References

1. Dejaco C, Ramiro S, Duftner C, Besson FL, Bley TA, Blockmans D, et al. EULAR recommendations for the use of imaging in large vessel vasculitis in clinical practice. Ann Rheum Dis. 2018;77(5):636-43

2. Duftner C, Dejaco C, Sepriano A, Falzon L, Schmidt WA, Ramiro S. Imaging in diagnosis, outcome prediction and monitoring of large vessel vasculitis: a systematic literature review and meta-analysis informing the EULAR recommendations. RMD Open. 2018;4(1):e000612.

3. Chrysidis S, Duftner C, Dejaco C, Schafer VS, Ramiro S, Carrara G, et al. Definitions and reliability assessment of elementary ultrasound lesions in giant cell arteritis: a study from the OMERACT Large Vessel Vasculitis Ultrasound Working Group. RMD Open. 2018;4(1):e000598.

4. Schafer VS, Juche A, Ramiro S, Krause A, Schmidt WA. Ultrasound cut-off values for intima-media thickness of temporal, facial and axillary arteries in giant cell arteritis. Rheumatology (Oxford). 2017;56(9):1632.

5. Diamantopoulos AP, Haugeberg G, Lindland A, Myklebust G. The fast-track ultrasound clinic for early diagnosis of giant cell arteritis significantly reduces permanent visual impairment: towards a more effective strategy to improve clinical outcome in giant cell arteritis? Rheumatology (Oxford). 2015.

6. Patil P, Williams M, Maw WW, Achilleos K, Elsideeg S, Dejaco C, et al. Fast track pathway reduces sight loss in giant cell arteritis: results of a longitudinal observational cohort study. Clin Exp Rheumatol. 2015;33(2 Suppl 89):S-103–6.

7. Diamantopoulos A, Haaversen AB. 085. The anteromedial ultrasound examination of the large supraaortic vessels identifies higher rates of large vessel involvement than previous reported in patients with giant cell arteritis. Rheumatology. 2019;58 Suppl 2:kez058.25.

8. Haaversen AB HV, Nabizadeh S, Slagsvold A, Diamantopoulos AP. Ultrasound to monitor treatment response in large vessel giant cell arteritis. Arthritis Rheumatol. 2019;71.

9. Touboul PJ, Hennerici MG, Meairs S, Adams H, Amarenco P, Bornstein N, et al. Mannheim carotid intima-media thickness and plaque consensus (2004–2006–2011). An update on behalf of the advisory board of the 3rd, 4th and 5th watching the risk symposia, at the 13th, 15th and 20th European Stroke Conferences, Mannheim, Germany, 2004, Brussels, Belgium, 2006, and Hamburg, Germany, 2011. Cerebrovascular diseases. 2012;34(4):290–6.

10. Terslev L, Diamantopoulos AP, Dohn UM, Schmidt WA, Torp-Pedersen S. Settings and artefacts relevant for Doppler ultrasound in large vessel vasculitis. Arthritis Res Ther. 2017;19(1):167.

11. Schafer VS, Chrysidis S, Dejaco C, Duftner C, Iagnocco A, Bruyn GA, et al. Assessing Vasculitis in Giant Cell Arteritis by Ultrasound: Results of OMERACT Patient-based Reliability Exercises. J Rheumatol. 2018;45(9):1289–95.

12. Aschwanden M, Daikeler T, Kesten F, Baldi T, Benz D, Tyndall A, et al. Temporal artery compression sign–a novel ultrasound finding for the diagnosis of giant cell arteritis. Ultraschall Med. 2013;34(1):47–50.

13. Fernandez-Fernandez E, Monjo-Henry I, Bonilla G, Plasencia C, Miranda-Carus ME, Balsa A, et al. False positives in the ultrasound diagnosis of giant cell arteritis: some diseases can also show the halo sign. Rheumatology (Oxford). 2020.

14. Diamantopoulos AP, Haugeberg G, Hetland H, Soldal DM, Bie R, Myklebust G. The diagnostic value of color Doppler ultrasonography of temporal arteries and large vessels in giant cell arteritis: A consecutive case series. Arthritis care & research. 2013.

15. Chrysidis S, Lewinski M, Schmidt WA. Temporal arteritis with ultrasound halo sign in eosinophilic granulomatosis with polyangiitis. Rheumatology (Oxford). 2019;58(11):2069–71.

16. Dasgupta B, Smith K, Khan AAS, Coath F, Wakefield RJ. Slope sign': a feature of large vessel vasculitis? Ann Rheum Dis. 2019;78(12):1738.

17. Milchert M, Brzosko M, Bull Haaversen A, Diamantopoulos AP. Correspondence to 'Slope sign': a feature of large vessel vasculitis? Ann Rheum Dis. 2019.

18. Gribbons KB, Ponte C, Carette S, Craven A, Cuthbertson D, Hoffman GS, et al. Patterns of Arterial Disease in Takayasu's Arteritis and Giant Cell Arteritis. Arthritis care & research. 2019.

19. De Miguel E, Beltran LM, Monjo I, Deodati F, Schmidt WA, Garcia-Puig J. Atherosclerosis as a potential pitfall in the diagnosis of giant cell arteritis. Rheumatology (Oxford). 2018;57(2):318–21.

The Salivary Glands

Iustina Janță

Patient Position

For the evaluation of major salivary glands (illustration 1), the patient is supine, with the neck hyperextended and the head turned to the opposite site.

Illustration 1 Anatomical diagram of salivary glands

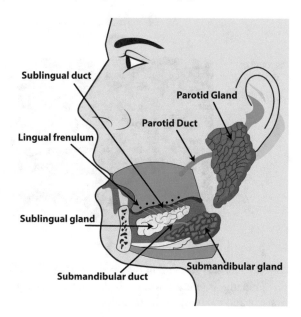

I. Janță (✉)
University Hospital Valladolid, Valladolid, Spain
e-mail: iustinajanta@yahoo.com

Fig. 1 Patient position
and probe position
(starting point) for the
longitudinal evaluation of the
submandibular gland

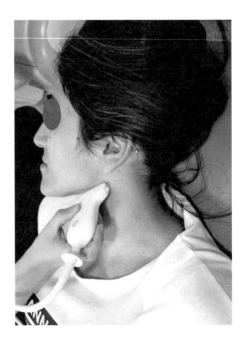

Fig. 2 Longitudinal view of
the submandibular gland

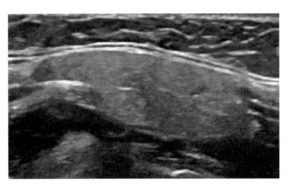

The *submandibular gland* is situated in the posterior part of the submandibular triangle. The submandibular triangle is formed by the anterior and posterior bellies of the digastric muscle and the body of the mandible.

For the evaluation of the submandibular gland (Illustration 2), the starting point is with the probe in longitudinal, parallel to the inferior aspect of the midpoint of the mandibular body (Figs. 1, 2). Then the probe is swept distally and medially for the evaluation of the entirely glandular parenchyma. Then the probe is changed to transverse and is swept from the anterior to posterior (Fig. 3). The submandibular

Fig. 3 Transverse view of
the submandibular gland

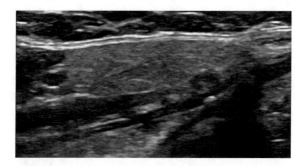

Fig. 4 Longitudinal view
of the submandibular
gland showing the facial
artery (arrow) between the
submandibular and parotid
glands

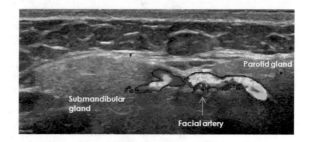

gland can be connected with the parotid gland, and the facial artery may be used
as a landmark between the two glands. Then, the facial artery may cross the submandibular gland parenchyma (Fig. 4).

Illustration 2 Anatomical diagram of submandibular gland

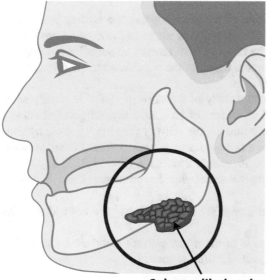

Submandibular gland

The *parotid gland (illustration 3)* is situated in the retromadibular fossa, anterior to the ear and sternocleidomastoid muscle. The superficial lobe covers partially the ramus of the mandible. Some parts of the deep lobe may be impossible to evaluate because the acoustic shadow of the mandibular ramus. The border between the superficial and the deep lobules is considered the plane that includes the facial nerve; as this nerve is not easily seen on ultrasound, the retromandibular vein (located above the trunk of the facial nerve) can be used as a landmark.

Illustration 3 Anatomical diagram of parotid gland

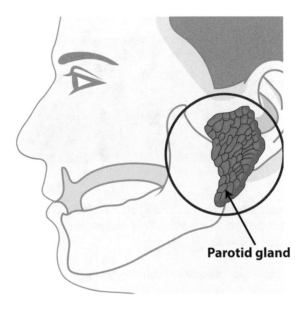

Parotid gland

For the evaluation of the parotid gland, the starting point is with the probe in longitudinal, from the mandibular ramus to the mastoid process (Figs. 5, 6). From this point the probe is swept from anterior to posterior. Then the probe is changed to transverse, from the tragus to the mandibular angle (Figs. 7, 8) and swept from proximal to distal.

The normal echogenicity of the salivary glands is usually compared to that of the thyroid gland or, in case of an altered thyroid gland, it could be compared to that of the adjacent muscle, the salivary gland being more hyperechoic. Both salivary glands have a homogeneous pattern. Intraglandular or periglandular lymph nodes can be seen in normal conditions (Fig. 9). It is important to evaluate the aspect of the lymph nodule with the presence of the hyperechoic hilum with Doppler signal.

The sublingual glands are very small, and are not useful in the assessment of Sjögren's syndrome.

For the evaluation of the major salivary glands, a linear probe, usually with a frequency between 10–15 MHz is needed.

Fig. 5 Patient position
and probe position (starting
point) for the longitudinal
evaluation of the parotid
gland

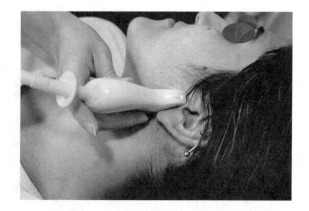

Fig. 6 Longitudinal view
of the parotid gland. *
retromandibular vein

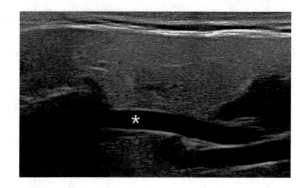

Fig. 7 Patient position and
probe position (starting point)
for the transverse evaluation
of the parotid gland

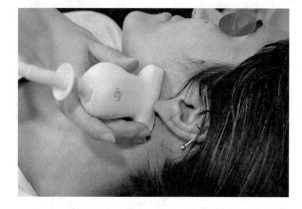

Fig. 8 Transverse view of
the parotid gland

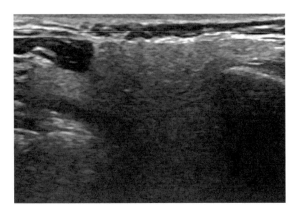

Fig. 9 Longitudinal view of
the parotid gland showing a
normal lymph nodule (arrow)

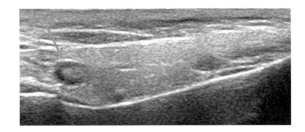

Pathology

Several salivary gland pathologies, acute (e.g. suppurate or obstructive sialadenitis) or chronic (e.g. Sjögren's syndrome, sarcoidosis, tuberculosis) can be evaluated by ultrasound. This chapter will focus on changes due to Sjögren's syndrome.

The Sjögren's is a chronic autoimmune disease that is characterised by a lymphocytic infiltration and destruction of the lachrymal and salivary glands. More than a half of the patients present also systemic involvement (e.g. pulmonary, neurological, renal or haematological). However, the symptomatology secondary to the destruction of salivary and lacrimal glands remain the principal manifestations of this disease.

Diagnostic of primary Sjögren's is made taking into account several clinical signs and symptoms, demonstration of salivary gland involvement and autoantibody testing. The current methods for the evaluation of salivary gland function and structure include salivary flow measurement, sialography, scintigraphy, minor salivary gland biopsy and MRI. Since the last decade of the last century, ultrasound was found to have specific changes in primary Sjögren's. Ultrasound has the advantages of being a fast, repetitive, non-invasive and non-irradiating technique. Thus, ultrasound is considered a valuable tool in the assessment of patients with Sjögren's.

Usually, both submandibular and parotid glands are evaluated by ultrasound. In Sjögren's the involvement of the salivary gland is bilateral and symmetrical.

Fig. 10 Longitudinal
view of the submandibular
gland showing abnormal
echogenicity

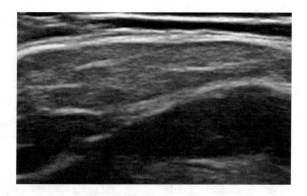

Fig. 11 Longitudinal view
of the submandibular gland
showing a moderate to high
heterogeneity of the glandular
parenchyma

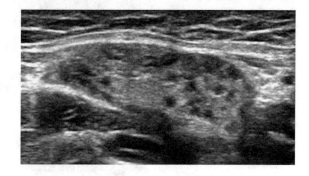

The main aspects that are assessed are the echogenicity and the homogeneity of glandular parenchyma. Other changes include the size of the salivary gland, the visibility of the posterior border, the presence of calcifications, hyperechoic bands, hypoechoic/anechoic areas and abnormal lymph nodes.

There are several scores developed to assess the involvement of salivary glands in Sjögren's. All of them include the assessment of echogenicity and homogeneity, the other features being included variably. The echogenicity is usually evaluated as normal or abnormal (Fig. 10). The heterogeneity is defined as the presence of hypoechoic/anechoic areas [1]. It has been evaluated on a semi quantitative scale form grade 0 (normal) to grade 2 to 4 (marked), depending on the score (Figs. 11–15). In the majority of the studies, a mild heterogeneity (grade 1) was considered within the normal variability (Fig. 16).

The usefulness of salivary gland US has been demonstrated for diagnostic purposes in several studies. A pooled sensitivity and sensibility of 69% and 92%, respectively, was found in a systematic review of 29 studies [2]. Furthermore, a recent study showed a good absolute agreement between salivary gland ultrasound and parotid and labial biopsy (i.e. 83% and 79%, respectively), with also a good sensitivity and specificity [3]. Another study found a significant relation between the abnormal salivary gland ultrasound and the presence of autoimmunity, the ESSDAI (EULAR Sjögren's Syndrome Disease Activity Index) value and

Fig. 12 Longitudinal view of the parotid gland showing a moderate heterogeneity of the glandular parenchyma

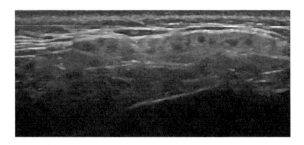

Fig. 13 Longitudinal view of the submandibular gland showing a high heterogeneity of the glandular parenchyma

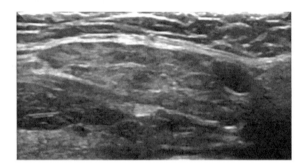

Fig. 14 Longitudinal view of the submandibular gland showing a moderate to high heterogeneity of the glandular parenchyma

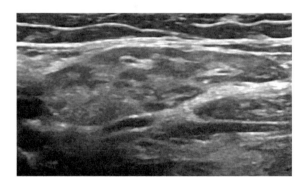

the presence of systemic disease, together with a higher risk markers of lymphoma (i.e. parotid enlargement, skin vasculitis and blood CD4 + T cells).

However, for the moment, there is not enough data to support the salivary gland ultrasound for monitory and prognostic purposes. This is mainly because of the difficulty in differentiating between inflammatory and chronic, fibrotic damages. Nevertheless, there are two studies investigating the responsiveness of salivary gland ultrasound in patients treated with rituximab, compared with placebo (TEARS and TRACTISS studies [4, 5]). The results of these two studies where not consistent; although in both studies improvement of salivary glands ultrasound was observed, in the first one, improvement in parotid gland echostructure was observed, while in the second one, improvement was due to the visibility of the salivary gland posterior border.

Fig. 15 Longitudinal view of the parotid gland showing a moderate heterogeneity of the glandular parenchyma

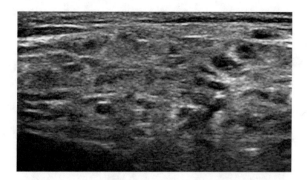

Fig. 16 Longitudinal view of the parotid gland showing a mild heterogeneity of the glandular parenchyma

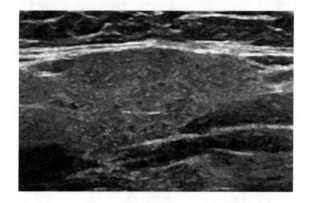

In conclusion, salivary gland ultrasound is a valuable tool in the diagnostic of patients with Sjögren's, the heterogeneity of glandular parenchyma being the most characteristic feature.

References

1. Theander E, Mandl T. Primary Sjögren's syndrome: diagnostic and prognostic value of salivary gland ultrasonography using a simplified scoring system. Arthritis Care Res. 2014;66:1102–7.
2. Delli K, Dijkstra P, Stel A, Bootsma H, Vissink A, Spijkervet F. Diagnostic properties of ultrasound of major salivary glands in Sjögren's syndrome: a meta-analysis. Oral Dis. 2015;21:792–800.
3. Mossel E, Delli K, van Nimwegen JF, et al. Ann Rheum Dis. 2017;76:1883–9.
4. Fisher BA, Everett CC, Rout J, et al. Effect of rituximab on a salivary gland ultrasound score in primary Sjögren's syndrome: results of the TRACTISS randomised double-blind multicentre substudy. Ann Rheum Dis. 2018;77:412–6.
5. Jousse-Joulin S, Devauchelle-Pensec V, Cornec D, et al. Brief report: Ultrasonographic assessment of salivary gland response to rituximab in Primary Sjögren's syndrome. Arthritis Rheumatol. 2015;67:1623–8.

Lung Ultrasound

Juan Carlos Nieto-González

Introduction

Lung ultrasound (LUS) has been used since the end of the 20th century to assess the presence of pulmonary oedema and pneumothorax [1]. Nowadays, the improvement of the US machines has allowed to increase the quality of the images and the usefulness of US in the assessment of the lung. LUS is frequently used in intensive care units, pulmonology and cardiology to assess pulmonary oedema (of whatever origin) and pneumothorax, but since the beginning of the 21st century LUS has been also used in the assessment of connective tissue diseases, specially systemic sclerosis (SSc), to assess interstitial lung diseases (ILD).

Lung Ultrasound Findings

Due to the air inside the lungs, LUS cannot usually assess the parenchyma of the lung [2]. However, when pneumonia takes place in the peripheral area of the lung, when there is pleuritis, ILD or a pneumothorax, LUS has shown to be very helpful in the assessment of the lung.

Normal LUS shows a hyperechoic line, moving with the breath, and regular and parallel hyperechoic reflections ('A' lines) deep to the pleura (Fig. 1). 'A' lines are a normal artefact of the pleura and should not be considered pathologic.

As already mentioned, in rheumatology the use of LUS is more recent and mainly focused on the assessment of ILD in SSc [3, 4]. Both, pulmonary oedema and ILD produce similar findings when assessed by LUS, comet tail or 'B' line artefacts, can be seen in the pulmonary pleura. Comet tail or 'B' line artefacts

J. C. Nieto-González (✉)
Hospital General Universitario Gregorio Marañón, Madrid, Spain
e-mail: Juancarlos.nietog@gmail.com

© The Author(s), under exclusive license to Springer Nature Switzerland AG 2021   247
Q. Akram and S. Basu (eds.), *Ultrasound in Rheumatology*,
https://doi.org/10.1007/978-3-030-68659-8_10

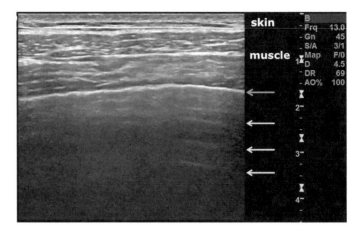

Fig. 1 Normal transverse LUS. Blue arrow: Pleura; Yellow arrows: 'A' lines

are hyperechoic lines perpendicular to and going down from the pleura (Fig. 2a). Usually, 'B' lines can be detected on its own or spread along the pleura but sometimes a number of 'B' lines are very close to each other giving a wide band image (Fig. 2b).

LUS also allows the detection of pleural irregularities, that together with 'B' lines have the same sensitivity than a high-resolution computerized tomography (HRCT) but pleural irregularities are more specific for ILD. Pleural irregularities can be seen as a thickening of the pleura and pleural defects that move with the breath (Fig. 2c).

How to Perform a LUS Examination

The LUS can be done with convex or linear probes, with a frequency range from 8 to 13 MHz, however, the authors recommend a linear probe with a 12–13 MHz frequency.

The patient could be laying down on the table in supine position or sitting on a stool. We should assess the intercostal spaces in the anterior and posterior thoracic wall [5]. (Illustration 1). The LUS assessment could be performed in a longitudinal (Fig. 3a) and in a transverse view (Fig. 3b). The longitudinal view shows the cortical of the ribs and in between allows detecting the pulmonary pleura. The transverse view shows the intercostal space, avoiding the cortical bone of the ribs.

The transverse view is preferred because it is possible to assess a larger part of the pleura, with the exception of the area of costal cartilage in the anterior thoracic wall (Fig. 3c).

The anterior thoracic wall examination should include the second to fifth intercostal spaces on the right side and from the second to fourth on the left side (Fig.

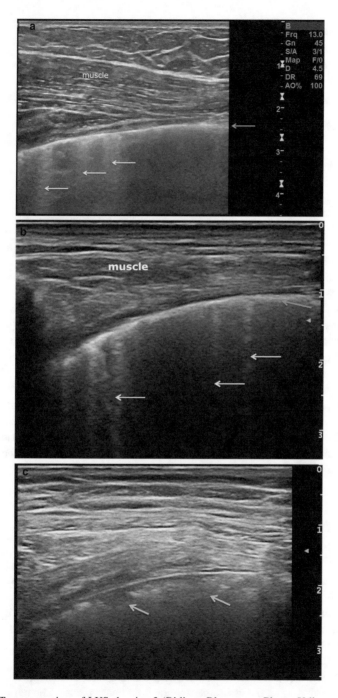

Fig. 2 a. Transverse view of LUS showing 3 'B' lines. Blue arrow: Pleura; Yellow arrows: 'B' lines. **b**. Transverse view of LUS showing 2 isolated 'B' lines on the right and 3 close 'B' lines on the left. Blue arrow: Pleura; Yellow arrows: 'B' lines. **c**. Transverse view of LUS showing pleural irregularities. Green arrows: pleural irregularities

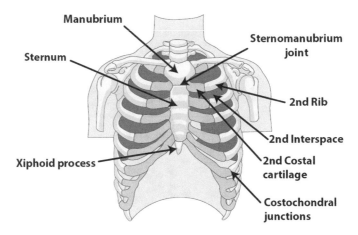

Illustration 1 Anatomical demonstration of the thorax. Figure commissioned by Dr Akram and printed with permission from Unzag Designs

4a and b). The posterior thoracic wall examination should include the paravertebral spaces from the seventh cervical vertebrae to the end of the lung (9th or 10th dorsal vertebrae) (Fig. 4c and d). In the last posterior spaces the intercostal space should be completely assessed from the paravertebral to the axillary area.

The main limitation of LUS is that it's time-consuming, taking around 20–30 minutes to perform a complete LUS examination. However, some authors have proposed a reduced LUS examination that maintains a good sensitivity and specificity but takes only 8.5 min to perform [6]. The reduced examination includes the bilateral assessment of the fourth midclavicular and axillar intercostal spaces in the anterior thoracic wall, the paravertebral space of the fourth posterior intercostal space and the complete assessment of the eight posterior intercostal spaces.

How to Interpret LUS

LUS has a good intra- and interobserver reliability (k: > 0.8). LUS is also very sensitive and specific (with an almost 100% of negative predictive value) for the detection of ILD in SSc. These characteristics make LUS a perfect tool for the screening of early ILD in connective tissue diseases, especially in SSc [7]. Moreover, the correlation between LUS and HRCT in detecting ILD is very high, with a concordance of an 83% [7, 8]. Some authors also showed a correlation between 'B' lines and a worse DLCO and capillaroscopy findings [8].

The presence of a few 'B' lines (less than 6 in the complete examination) should be a normal finding in the assessment of the pulmonary pleura. The cut-off point to consider it being pathological is detecting 10 'B' lines (sensitivity of 96,3% and a specificity of 92,3%), that should always be confirmed with a HRCT [9]. There is

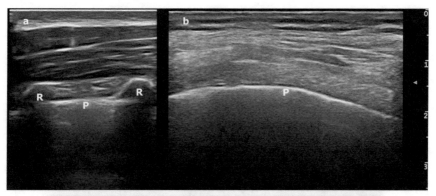

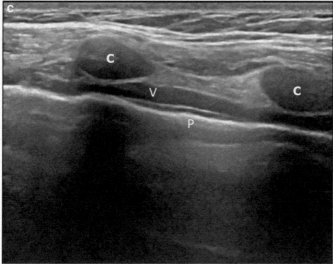

Fig. 3 Transverse Longitudinal (**a**) and longitudinal transverse (**b**) views of a normal LUS. R: Rib; P: Pleura. **c**. Longitudinal view LUS at the level of the costal cartilages. C: cartilage; V: thoracic vein; P: pleura

no agreement when detecting 6 to 10 'B' lines and this should be considered altogether with clinical symptoms and DLCO.

Inflammatory myopathies produce a higher number and larger pleural irregularities, together with 'B' lines, which is a very specific finding for these diseases (Fig. 5).

In rheumatoid arthritis, ILD could appear in 25–30% of patients, being symptomatic less than 5%. In some cases LUS can help in the early diagnosis diagnosis by detecting 'B' lines with usually normal pleural aspect (Fig. 6). Similar images can be detected in connective tissue diseases.

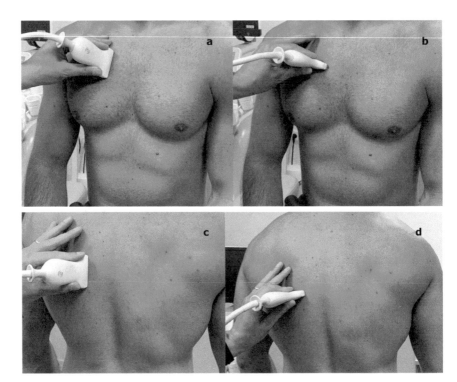

Fig. 4 Anterior and posterior examination of the thoracic wall using a longitudinal (**a** and **c**) and transverse approach (**b** and **d**). Note that the probe is transverse to the intercostal space and should be placed a bit oblique to get the correct image

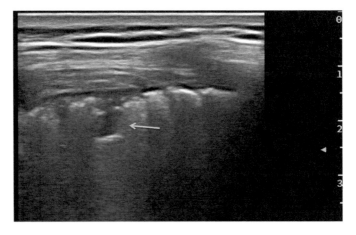

Fig. 5 Transverse LUS of a patient with a MDA-5 myopathy showing a great number of pleural irregularities. Green arrow: big pleural irregularity

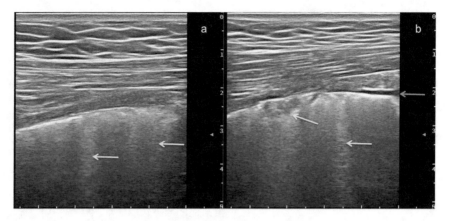

Fig. 6 56 years old male diagnosed with rheumatoid arthritis and chronic cough since 6 months ago. Transverse image of basal right lung shows 'B' lines (**a**) and pleurial irregularities (**b**). Blue arrow: Pleura; Yellow arrows: 'B' lines; Green arrow: pleural irregulatiry

Take-Home Messages

-LUS is easy to perform, reliable but can be time-consuming. A shorter and more succint examination has been proposed by some.

-The LUS assessment should include the anterior and posterior thoracic walls.

-'B' lines and pleural irregularities are the main findings that should be assessed with LUS.

-LUS is very useful in the screening of ILD thanks to it's high sensitivity and high negative predictive value. However LUS does not exclude the need to perform a HRCT in highly suspected patients.

References

1. Lichtenstein D, Mézière G, Biderman P, et al. The comet-tail artifac. An ultrasound sign of alveolar-interstitial syndrome. Am J Respir Crit Care Med. 1997;156:1640–6.
2. Wang Y, Gargani L, Barskova T, et al. Usefulness of lung ultrasound B-lines in connective tissue disease-associated interstitial lun disease: a literature review. Arthritis Res Ther. 2017;19:206.
3. Gargani L, Doveri M, D'Errico L, et al. Ultrasound lung comets in systemic sclerosis: a chest sonography hallmark of pulmonary interstitial fibrosis. Rheumatology (Oxford) 2009;48:1382–7.
4. Ferro F, Delle SA. The use of ultrasound for assessing interstitial lung involvement in connective tissue diseases. Clin Exp Rheumatol. 2018;36:S165–70.
5. Gargani L, Volpicelli G. How I do it: lung ultrasound. Cardiovascular Ultrasound. 2014;12:25.

6. Gutierrez M, Salaffi F, Carotti M, et al. Utility of a simplified ultrasound assessment to assess interstitial pulmonary fibrosis in connective tissue disorders- preliminary results. Arthritis Res Ther. 2011;13:R134.
7. Barskova T, Gargani L, Guiducci S, et al. Lung ultrasound for the screening of interstitial lung disease in very early systemic sclerosis. Ann Rheum Dis. 2013;72:390–5.
8. Gigante A, Rossi Fanelli F, Lucci S, et al. Lung ultrasound in systemic sclerosis: correlation with high-resolution computed tomography, pulmonary function tests and clinical variables of disease. Intern Emerg Med. 2016;11:213–7.
9. Gargani L, Doveri M, D'Errico L, et al. Ultrasound lung comets in systemic sclerosis: a chest sonography hallmark of pulmonary interstitial fibrosis. Rheumatology (Oxford). 2009;48:1382–7.

Index

© The Editor(s) (if applicable) and The Author(s), under exclusive license to Springer
Nature Switzerland AG 2021
Q. Akram and S. Basu (eds.), *Ultrasound in Rheumatology*,
https://doi.org/10.1007/978-3-030-68659-8

Printed in the United States
by Baker & Taylor Publisher Services